ACCOUNTABLE

The Baylor Scott & White Quality Alliance
Accountable Care Journey

The transformation of the U.S. health care delivery system to one based upon value and accountability is one of the compelling stories of our time. To undertake this transformation requires building a culture of accountability. And that requires leadership. This compelling book tells the story of how an already renowned institution built an organization to deliver better care for the patients it serves. Others attempting this task will find this invaluable.

Joe Cunningham, MD
Managing Director
Santé Ventures

This is the definitive primer and 'user's guide' for health care executives and operating leaders who are designing, developing, or deploying an ACO. It is equally valuable for industry stakeholders as they partner and collaborate with ACOs. Invaluable insights, strategies, and tactics from an industry pioneer that will enable you to move forward effectively and efficiently.

Michael Weintraub
President & CEO
Optum Analytics

This is a very complete, yet concise story of the Baylor Scott & White Health accountable care journey. This book is a must read for any health care system leader or physician leader who is developing or serving as a leader in an accountable care organization.

Paul B. Convery, MD, MMM
Clinical Professor of Healthcare Leadership & Management
Naveen Jindal School of Management
University of Texas Dallas
Former Chief Medical Officer
Baylor Health Care System

In a time of consolidation and turmoil in health care, Couch and his colleagues provide a clear and concise game plan for bringing organizations together around real performance—improving outcomes and efficiency. This is a forward-looking yet practical book that touches on the full range of issues that come up in a typical day and a typical decade for emerging accountable care organizations. It is well-written, thoughtful, and credible—an important contribution.

Thomas H. Lee, MD
Chief Medical Officer
Press Ganey Associates, Inc.
Professor (Part Time)
Harvard Medical School

Most large health care organizations today are re-imagining the delivery of and payment for health care services. The Baylor Scott & White Quality Alliance (BSWQA) has actually started the process and is demonstrating impressive preliminary results. Texas Health Care is proud that many of our physicians are affiliated members of the BSWQA.

Larry Tatum, MD
President & CEO
Texas Health Care, P.L.L.C.

Accountable is nothing less than a clarion call for accelerating the transformation from provider-centric volume to patient-centric value in health care. The description of BSWQA's journey, which includes governance, care delivery innovations, process, staffing, and payment models, creates a readable and engaging "ACO primer" which is timely and unique. BSWQA's story represents a rare, honest "look under the hood" of what it takes to make an ACO and its tenets of population health actually happen—and in the near term. This book should be widely read for its leadership vision, practical perspective, and operational considerations applicable to every provider and delivery system. This "ACO parable in real life" has lessons for even the most established medical group or health system.

Michael Parkinson, MD, MPH, FACPM
Senior Medical Director of Health & Productivity
UPMC Health Plan

Dr. Couch and his colleagues provide a valuable resource for anyone seeking to understand accountable care and population health. The story of the Baylor Scott & White Quality Alliance's journey provides an excellent model with practical examples for others to learn from. This book is a must read for anyone whose organization is seeking to achieve the Triple Aim.

Gary Yates, MD
President
Sentara Quality Care Network
President
Healthcare Performance Improvement, LLC
Former Senior Vice President and Chief Medical Officer
Sentara Healthcare

It is increasingly difficult in health care to navigate a course between the competing interests of providing high-quality care for our community of patients and maintaining fiscal responsibility. Consumers must be able to afford quality medical care, and health systems must be able to provide it in a fiscally prudent manner. The Baylor Scott & White Quality Alliance is transforming its system and relationships with providers and setting a benchmark for other health systems to attain, including population health accountability and pay for performance. This book maps a pathway to successful implementation.

J. Lindsey Bradley, Jr., FACHE
President
Trinity Mother Frances Hospitals and Clinics

Dr. Couch and his team have upheld the profound Baylor Scott & White Health tradition of passionate leadership in Patient Care, Community Service, Education and Research through this new book outlining responsible disruptive innovation to take us to Value-Based Care. With the foundation of the Hippocratic Oath to the work of the Institute of Medicine to STEEEP (safe, timely, effective, efficient, equitable, patient-centered care), they chart a comprehensive, practical and personal journey for all of us in leadership, and those we serve, to replicate and scale. The Health Employer Exchange members will be enlightened and inspired to adapt it throughout our nation.

Stephanie S. McCutcheon
Innovation/Transformation Advisor
Health Employer Exchange

ACCOUNTABLE

The Baylor Scott & White Quality Alliance
Accountable Care Journey

Carl Couch, MD, MMM

Editors:
Briget da Graca, JD, MS
Kathleen M. Richter, MBA, MS, MFA
Jean Sullivan, MBA

Foreword by Lee B. Sacks, MD
Executive Vice President & Chief Medical Officer, Advocate Health Care

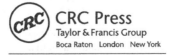

CRC Press
Taylor & Francis Group
Boca Raton   London   New York

CRC Press is an imprint of the
Taylor & Francis Group, an **informa** business
A PRODUCTIVITY PRESS BOOK

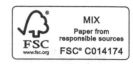

CRC Press
Taylor & Francis Group
6000 Broken Sound Parkway NW, Suite 300
Boca Raton, FL 33487-2742

© 2016 by Baylor White & Scott Health
CRC Press is an imprint of Taylor & Francis Group, an Informa business

Printed on acid-free paper
Version Date: 20151103

International Standard Book Number-13: 978-1-4987-4333-4 (Hardback)

Visit the Taylor & Francis Web site at
http://www.taylorandfrancis.com

and the CRC Press Web site at
http://www.crcpress.com

This book is dedicated to my daughter,
Dr. Kimberly McMillin, an *accountable* physician,
and to the many other physicians and professionals
who have chosen to hold themselves accountable
to transform health care in pursuit of the Triple Aim.

Contents

Foreword

November 1, 2015 marked the opening of the third annual enrollment period for the public exchanges under the Affordable Care Act (ACA), and was more than five and a half years after the ACA was signed into law by President Obama. Concurrent with the changes brought on by the ACA, there have been changing market forces driven by the Great Recession and the need for American businesses to compete in a global economy. The latter pressures will ensure that the dramatic changes occurring in the health care industry will continue regardless of the fate of the ACA after the 2016 election.

While Accountable Care Organizations (ACOs) were initially a Medicare demonstration project and were then authorized via the Center for Medicare and Medicaid Innovation under the ACA, they have proliferated in the commercial sector as health plans have tried to create incentives to reduce costs, and organized provider systems have sought aligned incentives to support achieving the Triple Aim of improving the patient experience of care, improving the health of populations, and reducing the per capita cost of health care.

ACO and population health management have become industry buzz words in the last several years that are being used to sell products, provide rationales for strategic initiatives, justify budget requests, and create burning platforms for change. It is important to define both terms so that they can be used consistently and understood by all. The book *Accountable* clearly defines both of these terms and makes them relevant for health care industry leaders.

Accountable is timely as it uses the journey of Baylor Scott
& White Quality Alliance (BSWQA) to define what an ACO is
and, even more important, helps to outline the accountabilities
for patients, providers, insurers, employers, and vendors that
are necessary for an ACO to be successful. BSWQA began its
journey in 2011 and over the next four years dealt with many
of the challenges that health care delivery systems across the
country are facing. Baylor Health Care System and Scott &
White Healthcare merged in 2013, combining two adjacent
delivery systems and adding a provider owned health plan.
BSWQA has a core of employed physicians, but also has a
large network of independent aligned physicians and serves
both an urban and a more rural service area that have a strong
history of using a fee-for-service payment model. Sharing the
BSWQA journey will provide insights that are relevant to all
health care delivery system leaders.

BSWQA is a work in progress. The book acknowledges
that for its journey to be successful, it will be disrupting its
legacy business model. Carl Couch, MD, MMM has shared
details of who, what, and why decisions have been made.
I would expect that BSWQA will make mid-course corrections
as it uses its data to continuously improve its processes, but
Accountable outlines a starting point for any organization
transforming into an ACO.

For anyone involved in their organization's efforts to
achieve the Triple Aim, *Accountable* can serve as both a
project plan and a check list to assure that all the necessary
infrastructure, aligned incentives, data transparency, and
leadership are in place for success. It will extend the impact
of BSWQA far beyond its service area, and allow many other
patients to benefit from the work that Dr. Couch has been
intimately involved with as president of BSWQA.

Lee B. Sacks, M.D.
Downers Grove, IL
November, 2015

Acknowledgements

It is a warm experience to reflect with acknowledgement and personal gratitude to God for the many life circumstances and individuals without whom this book would not have come together. Greatest of those in my personal career is my life's love, best friend, and counselor, Jo Anna Couch. Her guidance and coaching in my years spent in clinical practice and in physician leadership have always kept me grounded and on track, and her reflections on this book have made it far more understandable and readable.

My twenty-two years of professional association with Baylor Scott & White Health (BSWH) have gone by very quickly. That relationship, and in turn this book, could not have occurred without the steadfast leadership and support for continuous pursuit of quality from BSWH Chief Executive Officer Joel Allison, Executive Vice President and Chief Integrated Delivery Network Officer Gary Brock, Board members, and fellow physician and nursing leaders in our health care system. Dr. David Ballard, Chief Quality Officer of BSWH, President of the STEEEP Global Institute, and my colleague and partner in our mutual quality journey, has graciously sponsored the origin and completion of this work, lending me the support of his great editorial and literary team. This team includes Nanette Myers, whose project management and executive editorial oversight kept our team focused and on time and whose content advice was invaluable; Kathleen Richter, whose writing skills shaped many pages of the book and who helped to clarify complexity; Briget da Graca, for particular help in making the multiple legal requirements of accountable care coherent; Jean Sullivan, who provided key information and editorial support with regard to population health; and Alyssa Zarro, for her administrative and logistical assistance.

Many individuals generously contributed their professional expertise to the actual content of the book. These include my physician and nursing friends and colleagues, Drs. Dighton Packard, Cliff Fullerton, David Bragg, David Winter, Glen Ledbetter, Wendy Oberdick, Glen Couchman, Tiffany Berry, Michael Massey, Bob Probe, Brett Stauffer, Irving Prengler, and Dora Bradley. Valuable contributions were made by our talented Accountable Care Organization (ACO), Managed Care, and IT professionals, including Alyssa Endres, Becky Hall, Megan Harkey, Randy Hoffman, Nick Reddy, Deirdre Marek James, Jenny Reed, Brandon Pope, and Dianne Grussendorf. Health plan insights from Dr. Ken Phenow and Marinan Williams were most helpful. The entire dedicated and capable leadership team of Baylor Scott & White Quality Alliance has been vital in the building of a great ACO and the writing of this book. Among those, particular thanks goes to Sarah Gahm, Bill Roberts, Trent Hadley, and Blake Allison, and for their many hours spent in interviews and reviews of those notes and comments.

Special thanks also goes to in-house counsel John Buerkert, who has skillfully authored the chapter on legal and regulatory requirements in accountable care, as well as input from outside counsel firms Hutton and Williams and Norton Rose Fulbright. Dr. Wendy Oberdick has been particularly helpful for eloquent care coordination and physician performance comments as well as case illustrations.

My long-term colleague and executive assistant Diane Ford has kept me on track, facilitated communication, and skillfully manipulated schedules to allow the book to come together in a timely manner.

Finally, during a forty-year career in health care, I have been blessed to know and work with many physicians, nurses, executives, and other health professionals who have always held themselves *accountable* for the delivery of safe, timely, effective, efficient, equitable, and patient-centered care. For those great individuals who wake up each day passionate about making health care better for both the patients that we serve, and for those who serve those patients, and who share the fellowship of those of us who are intent on making that happen, I am very, very grateful. I am pleased that it is a growing fraternity, and one that will help to profoundly transform health care.

Carl E. Couch, MD, MMM

About the Author

Carl E. Couch, MD, MMM, FAAFP is a Board-Certified Family Physician, Diplomat of the American Board of Family Practice, and Fellow of the American Academy of Family Physicians. An active family physician for nearly 40 years, he founded Family Medical Center at Garland, Texas, the first group practice acquired by Baylor Health Care System in 1993.

Dr. Couch was a Founding Director and 13-year Chairman of the Board of HealthTexas Provider Network (HTPN), a multi specialty medical group comprising over 850 providers practicing in 250 care delivery sites across North Texas. He was also Founder and Executive Director of ABC Baylor (now called STEEEP Academy), the Baylor Scott & White Health (BSWH) training course on rapid-cycle quality improvement organized around the six domains of STEEEP care: safety, timeliness, efficacy, efficiency, equity, and patient centeredness. Dr. Couch served as Vice President of Health Care Improvement for Baylor Health Care System before it joined with Scott & White Healthcare in October 2013 to form BSWH. Additionally, Dr. Couch served as Co-Chairman of the quality-focused Best Care Committee from 2005 through 2011 and was Director of Physician Leadership training within BSWH for over eight years.

From 2011 through June 2015, Dr. Couch served as President of Baylor Scott & White Quality Alliance (BSWQA), a clinically integrated accountable care alliance of over

4,000 primary and specialty care physicians, 46 hospitals, 29 post-acute care facilities, retail pharmacy clinics, and other providers aligned with BSWH, the largest not-for-profit health care system in Texas.

Dr. Couch's interests as a physician leader include accountable care, physician group dynamics, group practice organization and function, physician compensation, physician leadership development, systematic quality improvement, and medical informatics. As the founding president of a large, successful accountable care organization (ACO), Dr. Couch is a recognized authority in ACO formation, development, and management.

Dr. Couch was an Alpha Omega Alpha graduate of the University of Florida College of Medicine, did his post-graduate training at Parkland Hospital in Dallas, and earned his Masters of Medical Management degree from Tulane University in New Orleans.

Dr. Couch has been happily married for 50 years to his wife, Jo Anna, who is a certified Personal Life and Executive Coach. They have two children, Kimberly McMillin, MD (who is also a Family Physician in HTPN and who has two daughters), and Dr. Christopher Couch, PhD, an executive of Lear Corporation in Detroit, who has a son and daughter. Dr. Couch enjoys golfing, boating, and travel, and is actively involved with his wife as co-teachers in adult education at Heights Baptist Church in Richardson, Texas, where he serves as a deacon.

Contributor List

Blake Allison, MS, FACHE
Chief Operating Officer
Baylor Scott & White
  Quality Alliance

Tiffany Berry, MD
Chief Patient Experience
  Officer
Baylor Scott & White Health
Vice President,
  Population Health
Baylor Scott & White
  Health-Central

**Dora Bradley, PhD,
RN-BC, FAAN**
Chief Clinical & Patient
  Learning Officer
Baylor Scott & White Health

David Bragg, MD
Medical Director of
  Clinical Integration
Baylor Scott & White
  Quality Alliance
Senior Vice President,
  Medical Informatics
HealthTexas Provider
  Network

John E. Buerkert, Jr., Esq.
Vice President & Assistant
  General Counsel
Baylor Scott & White Health

Glen Couchman, MD
Chief Medical Officer
Baylor Scott & White
  Health-Central

Alyssa Endres, MHA
Director, Strategic Initiatives
Baylor Scott & White
    Quality Alliance

Cliff Fullerton, MD, MSc
Chief Medical Officer
Baylor Scott & White
    Quality Alliance
Chief Officer for Population
    Health & Equity
Baylor Scott & White Health

Sarah Gahm, MHA
Senior Vice President & Chief
    Administrative Officer
Baylor Scott & White Quality
    Alliance & HealthTexas
    Provider Network

Dianne Grussendorf, MS
Senior Vice President,
    Managed Care
Baylor Scott & White Health

Trent Hadley, CPA, MSA
Manager, Healthcare
    Economics & Contract
    Performance
Baylor Scott & White
    Quality Alliance

Becky Hall
Vice President,
    Health & Wellness
Baylor Scott & White Health

Megan Harkey, MHA
Director, Strategic Initiatives
Baylor Scott & White
    Quality Alliance

Randolph Hoffman, MBA
Chief Financial Officer
Baylor Scott & White
    Quality Alliance

Thomas G. Ledbetter, MD
Chief Medical Officer
    & Vice President
    of Medical Affairs
Baylor Scott & White Medical
    Center-Waxahachie
Chief of Clinical Efficiency
HealthTexas Provider
    Network

Deirdre Marek James, MBA
Vice President,
    Project Implementation
Baylor Scott & White
    Quality Alliance

Michael Massey, MD
Vice President,
    Clinical Integration
Baylor Scott & White
    Quality Alliance

Wendy Oberdick, MD
Vice President, Network
    Performance
Baylor Scott & White
    Quality Alliance

Dighton Packard, MD
Chairman,
  Board of Managers
Baylor Scott & White
  Quality Alliance
Chief Medical Officer
Envision Health

**Ken Phenow, MD,
MPH**
Chief Medical Officer
Scott & White Health Plan

Brandon Pope, PhD
Director of Analytics
Baylor Scott & White
  Quality Alliance

**Irving Prengler, MD,
MBA**
Chief Medical Officer
Baylor Scott & White
  Health-North

Robert Probe, MD
Board of Trustees
Baylor Scott & White
  Holdings
Chairman
Scott & White
  Clinic Board of Directors
Chief of Staff
Scott & White
  Memorial Hospital

Nick Reddy, MBA
Senior Vice President,
  IS Investments
Baylor Scott & White Health

Jenny Reed, LCSW, ACM
Vice President,
  Comprehensive Care
  Management
Baylor Scott & White Health

**William L. Roberts,
MHA, CPA**
Senior Vice President
  & Chief Strategy Officer
Baylor Scott & White Health

**Brett Stauffer, MD,
MHS, FHM**
Vice President of Hospital
  Care Improvement
Baylor Scott & White Health

**Marinan Williams, MS,
FACHE, CMCE**
Interim CEO & President
Scott & White Health Plan

**F. David Winter, Jr., MD,
MSc, MACP**
President, Chairman,
  & Chief Clinical Officer
HealthTexas Provider
  Network

Introduction

Forming an accountable care organization (ACO) sounds relatively straightforward, but for an organization and its members to hold themselves *accountable* for transforming the way we deliver care, improve quality, reduce cost, and create a seamless, integrated care experience for patients is challenging. This book is meant to provide valuable insight into one organization's journey in developing an ACO. It details the experience of the Baylor Scott & White Quality Alliance (BSWQA), the ACO owned by Baylor Scott & White Health (BSWH), the largest not-for-profit health care system in Texas.

We begin from the question of why an organization like BSWH would form an ACO, and how it goes about meeting the relevant requirements and regulations and establishing the essential infrastructure for effective population health management and potential shared rewards. We then describe how BSWQA in particular and ACOs in general address accountability for transforming care delivery to achieve the three elements of the Triple Aim™ framework: improved experience of care, improved health for a population, and reduced cost per capita (Figure 1) [1, 2]. The Triple Aim Framework was developed by the Institute for Healthcare Improvement (IHI) in Cambridge, Massachusetts and is widely held today to be a national imperative for health care.

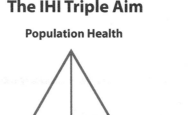

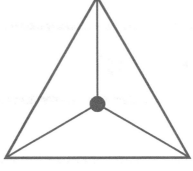

Figure 1 Triple Aim.

We will carefully discuss how BSWQA is attempting to improve quality, reduce cost, and better clinically integrate care. Additionally, we hope to seriously probe the concept of ***accountability*** for all of the stakeholders in our complex care system, and the important role of personal and organizational accountability in order to effectively and efficiently manage patient populations and achieve those aims. This book will raise questions and frame the actions and perspectives that participants in health care will have to modify in order to truly be accountable for achieving a high-quality, cost-effective, value-based care system. We devote a great deal of discussion to the "accountable" element of the ACO and how it might be deemed to be an essential driver of the many changes that need to take place within the health care system and for achieving the national imperatives outlined by the Triple Aim.

BSWQA was established in 2011 as part of the Baylor Health Care System (BHCS) "Vision 2020" strategy to become an accountable care delivery organization. Baylor Health Care System's board of directors envisioned the ACO as bringing together physicians (both employed and independent), hospitals, post–acute care, and other entities

CARE ACROSS THE
CONTINUUM

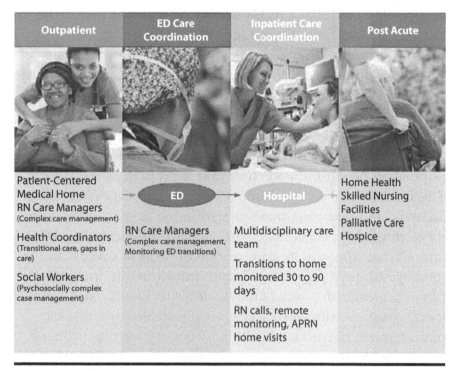

Outpatient	ED Care Coordination	Inpatient Care Coordination	Post Acute
Patient-Centered Medical Home RN Care Managers (Complex care management) Health Coordinators (Transitional care, gaps in care) Social Workers (Psychosocially complex case management)	**ED** RN Care Managers (Complex care management, Monitoring ED transitions)	**Hospital** Multidisciplinary care team Transitions to home monitored 30 to 90 days RN calls, remote monitoring, APRN home visits	Home Health Skilled Nursing Facilities Palliative Care Hospice

Figure 2   Continuum of Care.

along the continuum of care in an alliance with the mission of delivering the highest-quality, most cost-effective, and best coordinated care to the populations served [3]. In 2014, after Dallas–Fort Worth–based BHCS merged with Scott & White Healthcare (SWH) to form BSWH, BSWQA extended its mission and membership to the central Texas region. Today, it is composed of a network of more than 4,000 primary and specialty care physicians and 46 hospitals, 29 post–acute care facilities, retail pharmacy clinics, home health, and other providers throughout the care continuum (Figure 2).

The story of BSWQA's journey is of interest because
the organization grew out of a long history of success in
the fee-for-service environment, similar to the payment
system dominating much of the U.S. health care system.
It demonstrates that while such an environment does create
challenges for the transformation to the value-focused,
accountable model that ACOs are based on—particularly in
the way it historically encourages the volume-based delivery
of clinical care in discrete units composed of siloed specialties
[4]—those obstacles are not insurmountable.

It is widely recognized that it is difficult to manage what
cannot be measured. Holding ourselves accountable for the
quality and costs of care delivered while managing the health
of entire patient populations requires a well-established
population health infrastructure and appropriate governance.
The fundamental structure must facilitate the data collection,
analysis, and reporting necessary to measure outcomes, monitor performance, coordinate care, achieve physician buy-in,
and allocate appropriate care resources. Critical success factors
for establishing a population health infrastructure include
physician leadership, data analytic tools, evidence-based protocols, care coordination, access to affordable care, disease
management, preventive health services, and strong primary
care based in the patient-centered medical home (PCMH)
model [5]. These structures provide the framework for closing
care gaps, effectively coordinating care, and creating a truly
clinically integrated system. Clinical integration is a key success factor for accountable care and for managing the care
for complex patients. One only needs to be ill with multiple
chronic conditions to realize that health care continues to
be fragmented and that clinical integration in most systems
remains elusive [6].

A very important base for the successful development
of BSWQA was the employed physician organization
(HealthTexas Provider Network [HTPN]) as its fundamental
core. This mature employed physician entity laid a solid

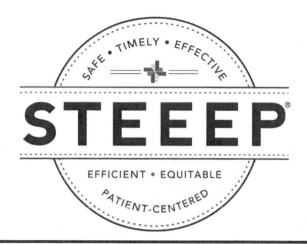

Figure 3   STEEEP care.

foundation from past and ongoing quality improvement
initiatives on which BSWQA could build. HTPN had been
making great strides in improving care delivery dating back
to 2001, when the organization began an alignment with
the Institute of Medicine's (IOM) six aims for health care
improvement, described as making care more safe, timely,
effective, efficient, equitable, and patient centered [7]. The IOM
stated, "Improvements require setting aims," a goal that was
carefully instilled in the culture of HTPN as well as the culture
of its counterpart, SWH clinics, for many years before the
merger. Demonstrating a true commitment to improving care
delivery, the IOM's six aims were rearranged into an acronym
and trademarked by BHCS as STEEEP® (safe, timely, effective,
efficient, equitable, and patient-centered) care (Figure 3).
The STEEEP acronym represents the "steep" climb from the
current state of the U.S. health care system to an ideal state
of health care delivery.

The STEEEP framework was an important driver of BSWH's
clinical transformation strategy and set the stage for BSWQA's
journey toward 21st-century medicine and achieving the
Triple Aim. Improvements made in all STEEEP domains laid
the groundwork for BSWQA's ability to extend beyond the six
aims and incorporate population health strategies by reducing

unnecessary variation, costs, waste, and errors, while simultaneously improving outcomes, access, and satisfaction.

BSWQA's successful formation of a population health infrastructure, and its capacity for care management and clinical integration, were built upon HTPN's accomplishments in becoming a high-performing health system. It drew on the physician organization's extensive experience in achieving patient satisfaction, installing a network-wide electronic health record (EHR), redesigning primary care sites to support the PCMH model, delivering reliable adult preventive health services, and managing chronic disease. This, together with the fact that the BSWQA leaders were selected from the past and present leaders within BSWH and HTPN, bringing with them an in-depth knowledge of the system's operation, strengths, and weaknesses relevant to the functioning of the ACO, were critical factors in how fast BSWQA was able to move from conception to reality.

Realizing that a successful ACO must be constructed to serve large numbers of patients, BSWQA, from its beginning, invited independent primary care and specialty physicians to join with the hospital-employed physicians in its formation. To date, many independent physicians have chosen to join and constitute more than 2,300 of the more than 4,000 physicians in BSWQA.

The relatively swift growth of BSWQA and subsequent positive results for improving population health outcomes over a short two-year period has been achieved by doing more than just relying on the framework established within existing hospitals and hospital-employed physician groups. Inclusion of such diverse participants creates a very different set of challenges. Can accountability be accomplished by a large, diverse physician group? What changes in perspective and practice are needed to achieve that? Could those changes disrupt existing practice patterns or economic self-interest?

BSWQA was designated by our health care system as the primary instrument through which BSWH can achieve the

Triple Aim for the populations we serve. Early data reported over the first two years of BSWQA's operation point to early success toward achieving this ambitious goal. BSWQA has established a dynamic population health infrastructure supported by a wide network of providers spanning the continuum of care who have contractually agreed to hold themselves *accountable* for the quality and costs of care provided to the more than 300,000 patients covered under the managed care agreements BSWQA holds as of October 1, 2015. Data from the two years for which BSWQA has been the preferred network for the 33,000-member BSWH North Texas division employee health plan show that BSWQA has built the capacity to effectively manage the health of plan enrollees. For example, three important population health outcomes show reductions: readmission rates, admissions per thousand, and total medical plan costs. But more important, we believe we are gradually growing our culture from one committed to quality to one also willing to hold ourselves accountable for the additional elements of the Triple Aim: managing the health of patient populations and reducing the cost of health care. We hope that our story is helpful to other providers and organizations considering embarking on, or engaged in developing, an ACO, in terms of both building the framework of factors critical to success and recognizing the cultural changes necessary for attaining *accountability*.

Chapter 1

Accountability

Main Points for Chapter

This chapter includes a discussion of:

- What it means to be accountable
- The importance of clinical integration: ensuring that the right patients receive the right care at the right time at the right place at the right cost and in a connected manner

Mr. B sits at his desk feeling troubled. At the age of 51, he has found himself diagnosed with multiple complex health conditions, leaving him feeling completely out of control of his health. The previous week he had experienced chest pains for a second time, but on attempting to contact his cardiologist, he had been told the cardiologist was out of town and the next available appointment was not for seven days. With the pressure in his chest building, he had gone to a nearby emergency department (ED), where he was promptly admitted. Cardiac catheterization by the on-call cardiologist identified a "blockage" that required insertion of a stent. His admitting lab tests revealed his blood sugar to be over 300 mg/dl—the highest it had ever been—and other tests revealed his lung function to be abnormal. Additionally, the catheterization identified a significant stenosis of his aortic valve, which needed surgical repair. However, the recommended valve repair needed to be delayed until his poor diabetic control was improved.

Two days later, Mr. B was discharged with a new cardiac stent and his blood sugar somewhat improved due to insulin initiation. At discharge he was presented with 30 minutes of instructions about managing his coronary artery disease, high blood sugar, and abnormal lung function, and was given a dozen sheets of printed discharge papers outlining these instructions. He was given prescriptions for insulin and syringes, several new medications (accompanied by alarming warnings about their potential side effects), a recommendation from the covering cardiologist to also see a cardiothoracic surgeon to schedule a valve repair and to see a pulmonary specialist, plus advice from the hospital to contact a primary care physician. The cardiologist advised a follow-up in one month. He hasn't received the hospital bills yet, but he is fairly certain that even with the help of his insurance coverage, the out-of-pocket costs for the hospital admission coupled with the costly new medications prescribed are going to strain his family's already limited household budget. With all of this new information to digest, he is not all that sure he remembers—or understands—the instructions he received about managing his conditions.

Reflecting on his current health circumstances, Mr. B admits to himself that he had not been diligent

about checking his blood sugar since being diagnosed with diabetes last year: the inconvenience of
checking his blood sugar at work by pricking his
finger frequently outweighed his endocrinologist's
warnings about its importance. He had also been
aware of some shortness of breath recently, but had
attributed those symptoms to being "out of shape,"
not the secondhand smoke from his wife's cigarettes.
He had not, however, expected anything to go
seriously wrong—at least not so soon.

Now phoning the primary care physician as
advised by the hospital, he is hoping to get an
appointment in a timely manner to begin the process
of resolving his health issues. He is disappointed to
find that the next available appointment for a new
patient is 45 days away. "This is why I rarely go to
a primary care physician. It seems to take forever
to get an appointment," he reflects. Thinking back
on previous office visits, he also recalls the redundancy of repeating the registration process and
health history review, followed by yet more rounds
of tests, some of them likely repeats of tests he had
just had during his hospital stay. "Don't these doctors
talk to each other? Doesn't anyone really know me?"
He wonders why health care is so complicated.

Mr. B is not an unusual patient in our health care system.
Physicians might label him unmotivated or noncompliant, and
while several of the specialists he saw in the hospital probably encouraged him to become engaged in his own health,
he doesn't know where to begin. Mr. B's multiple complex
conditions are causing him to miss work, leading his employer
to note that he is becoming less productive. Managing his
own health is overwhelming, leaving him confused and somewhat depressed. To most of his family and coworkers, he is
not himself. To objective professional observers, he appears

very off-track with limited likelihood of experiencing positive health outcomes in his near future.

Further, Mr. B's likely health care costs each year will approach many times the cost of a well-controlled diabetic with all coronary risk factors well controlled.

Mr. B's case provokes some important questions for the broader health care system to address:

1. Who should be *accountable* for Mr. B's care and outcomes?
2. How should a system of care ensure that the right patients receive the right care at the right time at the right place and at the right cost to prevent downward health trajectories such as what Mr. B is likely to experience?
3. How can we better engage patients like Mr. B in self-management of their complex health conditions so that they are more engaged, healthier, and more in control of their outcomes?

In most communities, today's health care systems cannot or do not achieve an ideal health care environment for Mr. B or patients like him. The questions above highlight the need for real health care system transformation to meet the needs of patients with multiple chronic diseases and limited understanding of and engagement in their health. Imagine a transformed system of health care that helps to prevent illness, allows convenient access to an experienced team of health care providers, and facilitates an established relationship with a primary care physician (PCP) anchored in PCMH. That medical home would be led by a PCP who is a "comprehensivist" whose primary responsibility is to manage and guide health needs across all care settings, utilize an EHR so that health information can be securely shared throughout a network of providers along the continuum of care, and offer treatment options based on evidence-based care. In such an ideal scenario, top-notch primary and specialty care would be coordinated by that medical home team. All of Mr. B's records would be available everywhere he went. His costs might be lower and true costs would be transparent. Redundancies might be reduced. His care would be safe, timely, effective, efficient, equitable, and very patient centered. What if Mr. B received care in the health system just described? Would he emerge as a healthier, more productive, and increasingly confident man and begin to experience an improved quality of life?

Few health care providers truly understand what it means to be a patient with complex conditions within poorly integrated health care systems. In fact, as physicians and other health professionals, we know exactly how to navigate the system and see "who we want," and because of our insider knowledge and relationships, more often than not our needs are met. From our vantage point, the system seems to run pretty well for us. However, most patients do not enjoy this reality. To those patients who might have multiple chronic diseases, mobility impairment, and poor social surroundings, the health care system seems perplexing, frustrating, unconnected, and difficult to navigate. Critics have said that we have constructed the health care system to serve providers rather than to serve patients.

Because the U.S. health care system is generally structured to encourage specialization, the physician workforce is more than two-thirds specialists [8]. Most specialty providers are siloed within their specialty, or center of excellence, and are absorbed in proficiently providing patients the particular aspect of care for which they are responsible. These specialty physicians largely are paid for visits and procedures. They are only partially exposed to the full picture of a patient with chronic disease visiting multiple practitioners and sites of care, and the need to prioritize and coordinate that care. Such a system may be effective in a generally healthy population, where the care primarily needed is in response to acute or discrete episodes of illness or injury. However, when attempting to care for patients and patient populations with a high (and growing) prevalence of chronic diseases that need to be managed simultaneously, the fragmented structure just described for Mr. B has proven to be highly ineffective and costly. He needs both a comprehensivist and multiple specialists working in close concert.

Our system is optimized for exceptional events and procedures, but not for complex disease management. Multiple authors note that the fragmented health care system in our country results in higher costs per capita with less than desirable outcomes than other developed countries [9, 10]. Extensive critiques of our system document that around 30% of the total cost of care is simply wasted [11].

Seamless patient navigation through the health care system—including care that happens between care episodes, between sites of care, and after care episodes—often determines much of the patient's outcome. Patients fall through the cracks between physicians, hospitals, and other providers far too often, resulting in suboptimal and costly outcomes. Clinical integration as supported by an accountable care structure is felt by many experts to be the most promising means for improving these patient transitions and ultimately achieving the three basic goals for improvement: improving the quality of care in any and all care settings, reducing the cost of care for the populations served, and clinically integrating care—particularly complex care—into a well-connected process *accountable* for better results [1]. Mr. B is unlikely to truly thrive without such a system.

Chapter 2

Why ACOs? How Can an Organization Produce Accountability?

Main Points for Chapter

This chapter includes a discussion of:

- What defines an accountable care organization
- Accountability for quality, cost, and clinical integration consistent with the Triple Aim
- How "value" in health care is defined in an accountable care world

The Accountable Care Organization

In an accountable care structure, physicians, hospitals, and others elect to come together and contractually agree to be jointly responsible and *accountable* for providing better care, better health, and better value to entire populations of patients, payers, and communities. They agree to collaborate, connect, follow evidence-based protocols, and be measured and compared in both quality and cost. Ideally, a physician-led interdisciplinary structure promotes a focus on managing both cost and quality and motivates health care stakeholders to work together, within disciplines and between disciplines, as they approach population health care and risk-related payment mechanisms. The ACO must significantly advance population health management and, if successful in the long term, will transform care delivery.

The ACO was conceptualized by Elliott Fisher, a physician and researcher at the Dartmouth Institute for Health Policy and Clinical Practice, and the term first appeared in print in a 2007 *Health Affairs* article proposing that freestanding hospitals and their affiliated physicians form virtual organizations that could be held accountable for the cost and quality of the full continuum of care delivered to their patients, improving the care those patients receive [12, 13]. ACOs rapidly began gaining traction following the establishment of the Medicare Shared Savings Program (MSSP) and the Medicare Pioneer ACO Program authorized in the Patient Protection and Affordable Care Act (ACA) in 2010 [14]. Today, there are more than 626 ACOs, focused on Medicare populations, commercial populations, or both [15].

While the ACO concept has evolved substantially since 2007, taking on a variety of forms, it has generally come to mean an "organization, virtual or real, that agrees to take on the responsibility for providing care for a particular population while achieving specified quality objectives and constraining costs" [13]. The providers within such organizations commit to being jointly *accountable* to patients and the ACO for the quality, efficiency, and cost of the health care provided. Steadily extending their presence nationwide [15], ACOs have come to be seen as one of the most promising strategies for achieving the Triple Aim [2]. Current ACO development focuses on achieving greater clinical integration across the

entire continuum of care, and that clinical integration must
be supported by true systemic change and meaningful reform
that expands coverage, improves quality and care coordination, rewards effective and efficient care, promotes innovation,
and helps control cost [16]. Clinical integration, as supported
by an ACO structure, offers a means for improving care for
patients like Mr. B, and from a broader perspective, hopefully
achieving the Triple Aim. Further, since the initial development
of ACOs, the fundamental role of primary care in the management of patients with complex conditions has been better
understood, and the importance of a robust primary care base
is increasingly appreciated. This has been a driving factor in
the proliferation of PCMHs, which help to close care gaps,
provide access, coordinate care more effectively, and ensure
a truly clinically integrated health care system [17].

What Does It Mean to Be Accountable?

In the world of medicine, the idea of accountability and being
accountable for patient care is not a new concept. Physicians
are familiar with being individually accountable for their
patients in the context of the traditional Hippocratic Oath
penned approximately 2,500 years ago. "The Hippocratic Oath
is one of the oldest binding documents in history. Written
in antiquity, its principles are held sacred by doctors to this
day: treat the sick to the best of one's ability, preserve patient
privacy, teach the secrets of medicine to the next generation,
and so on. 'The Oath of Hippocrates,' holds the American
Medical Association's Code of Medical Ethics (1996 edition),
'has remained in Western civilization as an expression of ideal
professional conduct for the physician'" [18]. Consider the
beginning of the oath (Figure 2.1): "I swear to fulfill, to the
best of my ability and judgment, this covenant."

"I swear." These powerful words commit the physician
to a very high performance standard that underlies today's

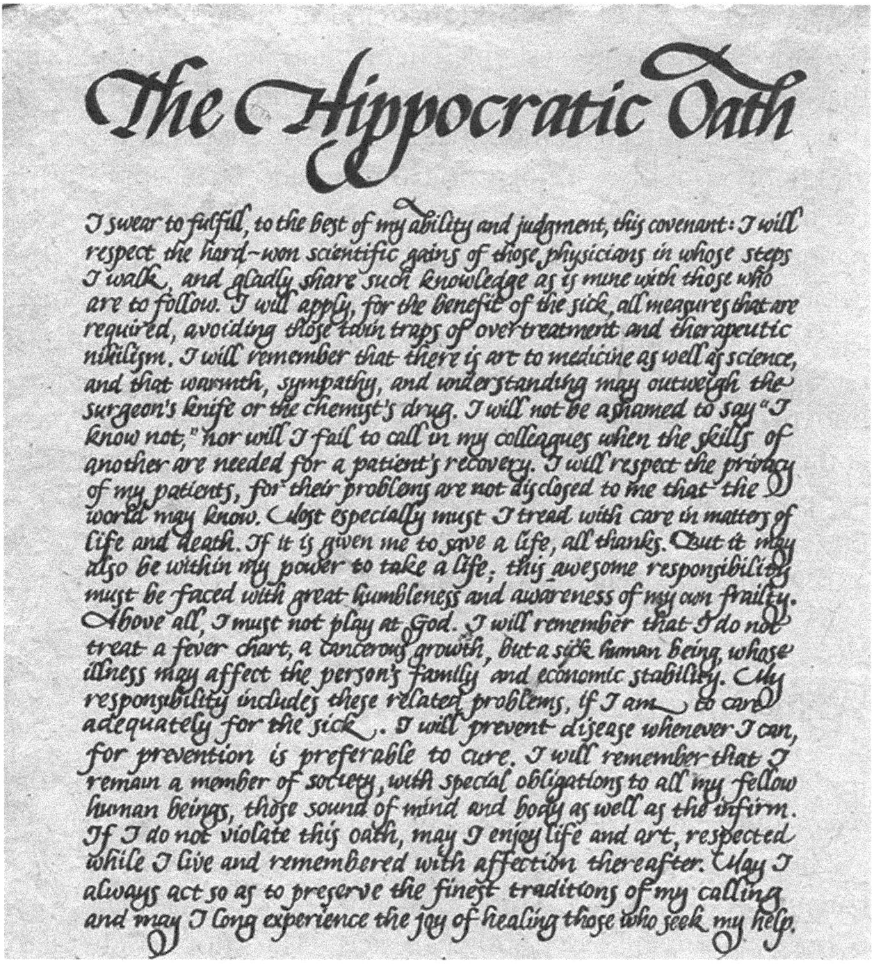

The Hippocratic Oath

I swear to fulfill, to the best of my ability and judgment, this covenant: I will respect the hard-won scientific gains of those physicians in whose steps I walk, and gladly share such knowledge as is mine with those who are to follow. I will apply, for the benefit of the sick, all measures that are required, avoiding those twin traps of overtreatment and therapeutic nihilism. I will remember that there is art to medicine as well as science, and that warmth, sympathy, and understanding may outweigh the surgeon's knife or the chemist's drug. I will not be ashamed to say "I know not," nor will I fail to call in my colleagues when the skills of another are needed for a patient's recovery. I will respect the privacy of my patients, for their problems are not disclosed to me that the world may know. Most especially must I tread with care in matters of life and death. If it is given me to save a life, all thanks. But it may also be within my power to take a life; this awesome responsibility must be faced with great humbleness and awareness of my own frailty. Above all, I must not play at God. I will remember that I do not treat a fever chart, a cancerous growth, but a sick human being, whose illness may affect the person's family and economic stability. My responsibility includes these related problems, if I am to care adequately for the sick. I will prevent disease whenever I can, for prevention is preferable to cure. I will remember that I remain a member of society, with special obligations to all my fellow human beings, those sound of mind and body as well as the infirm. If I do not violate this oath, may I enjoy life and art, respected while I live and remembered with affection thereafter. May I always act so as to preserve the finest traditions of my calling and may I long experience the joy of healing those who seek my help.

Figure 2.1 The Hippocratic Oath.

concepts of professionalism. Today, most graduating medical school students swear to some form of the oath, usually a modernized version. Indeed, oath taking in recent decades has risen to near uniformity, with just 24% of U.S. medical schools administering the oath in 1928 to nearly 100% today [18].

There are contrary viewpoints as to whether the Hippocratic Oath is relevant in today's world of 21st-century medicine, given the tremendous scientific, economic, political, social, and cultural changes present. After all, what does the Hippocratic Oath have to do with accountability centered on improving quality, managing entire patient populations, and reducing costs? In our current environment of increasing medical specialization, should physicians swear to a single oath? With governments and health care organizations sharing patient information as never before, how can a doctor solely maintain a patient's privacy? Many in the industry contend that while its original philosophy dates back to the Greeks, the Hippocratic Oath still continues to provide a road map for maximizing the patient experience and outcomes within the medical profession while also laying the groundwork for a future *accountable* care delivery system.

The Hippocratic Oath connotes a sense of "professional duty" taken at a critical time in the development of the physician as he or she passes from one stage of the journey (medical school) to the next stages of training and providing care. Rather than a legally binding oath, it serves as a sign of personal importance, commitment, and solemnity as physicians embark on echoing the essence of the Hippocratic Oath. The oath could be capsulized by such phrases as: "May I care for others as I would have them care for me," and "I will put my patients interest above my own." It can be argued that it is in this context that the ACO structure is formed based on individual provider commitment to voluntarily be *accountable* for achieving improved quality, enhanced patient experience, and reduced costs through clinical integration. By joining an ACO, physicians commit in principle and by contractual agreement to be accountable for these deliverables—a new commitment to very old values.

Breaking down a modernized version of the Hippocratic Oath, one might make additional statements that resonate with accountable care objectives that ACO providers are voluntarily committing to:

■ **Quality improvement:** "I will prevent disease whenever I can, for prevention is preferable to cure."

- **Enhanced patient experience:** "I will remember that I do not treat just a fever chart, or a cancerous growth, but a sick human being, whose illness may affect the person's family and economic stability." Clearly communicating with the patient using shared decision making, "I will deliver my care in the most patient-centered manner, trying to produce outcomes that matter to patients" [19].
- **Clinical integration:** "Even though I specialize in a certain field, I will participate and connect with those other care team members, always mindful that holistic care usually has best outcomes."
- **Cost:** "I will avoid costly nonbeneficial treatments and reduce waste, even waste I was previously paid for."

Accountability is broadly defined as having an obligation or willingness to accept responsibility or to account for one's actions [20] or, alternatively, having the obligation to answer questions regarding decisions or actions [21]. But a practical definition of accountability requires answering some questions: Accountable for what, accountable to whom, and accountable by whom? Answers can be generally grouped into three categories: performance (quality), financial (cost), and clinical integration. Additionally, attention to the greater social responsibility involved in overall health care cost and delivery will be kept in mind [21]. As such, in the specific context of health care organizations, accountability has been defined as "taking into account and responding to political, commercial, community, and clinical/patient interests and expectations" and "the process by which health leaders pursue the objectives of efficiency, quality, and access to meet the interests and expectations of these significant 'publics'" [22]. But while this definition answers the high-level question of what accountability means for an organization as a whole, it leaves open questions about the individuals who make up that organization. Who is responsible for specific aspects of health care delivery, such as decisions, policies, administration, governance, reporting, and ultimately answering for consequences of the care delivered? Are physicians to be solely responsible? What about hospitals and post–acute care providers? Should pharmaceutical manufacturers and device makers be accountable? And what is the role of patients themselves?

Care delivered to patients like Mr. B, who may have multiple comorbid conditions, is often complex, time-consuming, and costly, and it usually involves a variety of health care stakeholders (the patient, PCPs, specialty physicians, hospitals, payers and insurers, and post acute care providers and facilities), all of whom have potential to impact quality and cost outcomes. Also, beyond those stakeholders with direct involvement in the care Mr. B receives, what about stakeholders such as regulators and employers? Reforming an entire complex health care system and creating the infrastructure necessary to achieve better value for patients will certainly be a complex challenge. It will likely involve disruptive changes in existing business models, in clinical decision making, and in the routine actions of all health care stakeholders involved. If the accountable movement is successful, it will transform an entire industry. So let's break down the three accountable goals: quality, cost, and clinical integration.

Accountability for Quality

Most physicians and other health care providers have a strong professional desire to do their best to deliver quality care to their patients. But in 2001, when the IOM report *Crossing the Quality Chasm: A New Health System for the 21st Century* was released, the serious deficiency in health care quality was brought into the spotlight [7]. This report stunned the U.S. health care community with its findings and assertion that there is a chasm (not just a gap) between the health care system in place and what is needed to achieve optimal outcomes and establish and maintain a healthy population.

Other reports confirmed the IOM's findings of quality deficiencies in the U.S. health care system. For example, a 2003 RAND corporation study conducted in a random sample of adults living in 12 cities across the United States found that participants received only 55% of the recommended care [23]. Also as the 1999 IOM report *To Err Is Human* had already shown, care delivered to patients was too often unsafe [24]. Issues related to access to and timeliness of care were shown to be important targets for improving quality of care. Patient outcomes and reducing overall costs [25–27] were shown to be important, along with the need to establish systems of coordinated care to manage the increasingly prevalent chronic conditions like diabetes, chronic obstructive pulmonary disease (COPD), heart failure, asthma, and depression that are not amenable to the fragmented, siloed structure rendered by the acute care model around which the U.S. health care system was built [28]. Finally, there was recognition that patients' wishes and preferences often took a back seat during decisions about their care under a frequently paternalistic model of medicine [29, 30].

In the face of such overwhelming evidence of deficiencies in these important aspects of care delivery, quality measurement and improvement became high priorities. As a result, the six STEEEP domains are the areas on which many health care organizations including BSWH have focused. Progress has been made in some areas—for example, nationally there was a 63% reduction in central-line-associated bloodstream infection (CLABSI) incidence from 2001 to 2009; surgical infections have been reduced by standardizing preoperative antibiotics; errors have been reduced by preoperative surgical safety time-outs and checklists; and there has been an increase in the adoption of health information technology (HIT). But improvement in other areas, including patient-centeredness, iatrogenic adverse events, and the siloed education and practice of health care professionals, has been disappointingly slow or absent [31, 32]. The principle of *accountability* lies at the heart of driving further improvement and is being encouraged through a variety of reforms in the organization and financing of health care, including ACOs, value-based payments, and public reporting requirements.

HTPN offers a real-world example of how health care organizations can achieve significant improvements through action and accountability: From 2000 to 2006, HTPN increased the proportion of its adult primary care patients for whom the recommended preventive services were "completed or done" from below 50% to 86%. HTPN achieved this through a multi-pronged quality improvement strategy that incorporated transparent physician-level and practice-level performance data feedback, and by holding physicians *accountable* to their peers [33, 34]. Over a period of six years and in a patient population of 245,000, this level of improvement was estimated to have prevented 36 deaths and 97 incident cases of cancer, 420 coronary heart disease events (including 66 sudden deaths) and 118 strokes, 816 cases of influenza and pneumonia (including 24 hospital admissions), and 87 osteoporosis-related fractures [35]. HTPN has continued to measure and report performance on delivery of 11 recommended adult preventive health services and has held performance steady, with 87% of patients seen in a recent period being up-to-date on all of the services for which they are eligible, a percentage significantly higher than the national Healthcare Effectiveness Data Information System (HEDIS) benchmark [36].

This quality success story required a journey of strong leadership plus learning and implementing process improvements throughout the organization. Physicians had to learn to use team medicine and the accurate measurement and reporting of data to help them identify areas to improve. But most important, it required organizational *accountability* that acknowledged and systematically addressed a real quality deficit.

Accountability for Cost

The forces driving increases in health care costs seem relentless. Industry and demographic factors—such as rapidly changing technology, the aging population, and increasing prevalence of lifestyle-associated diseases—together with the health care system's traditional focus on treatment rather than prevention, and the dominance of the fee-for-service payment model, have helped to drive a high medical care inflation rate over the last ten years [37] (Figure 2.2). This cost curve exceeds the consumer price index and the gap continues to grow. For years, critics of the health care system have recognized that the rising cost of care is unsustainable and is caused by the provision of *too much* unnecessary or ineffective care, *too little* effective care (particularly in the areas of disease prevention and management), and *wrong care* [7, 38]. Under the fee-for-service reimbursement mechanism, however, health care providers and organizations have been paid generously despite—and, indeed, sometimes *because of*—these inefficiencies in care.

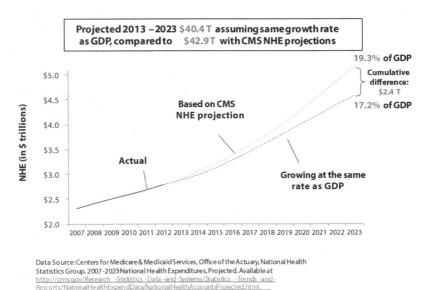

Data Source: Centers for Medicare & Medicaid Services, Office of the Actuary, National Health Statistics Group. 2007-2023 National Health Expenditures, Projected. Available at http://cms.gov/Research -Statistics -Data -and -Systems/Statistics -Trends -and- Reports/NationalHealthExpendData/NationalHealthAccountsProjected.html.

Figure 2.2 What if National Health Expenditures (NHE) grew at the same rate as GDP?

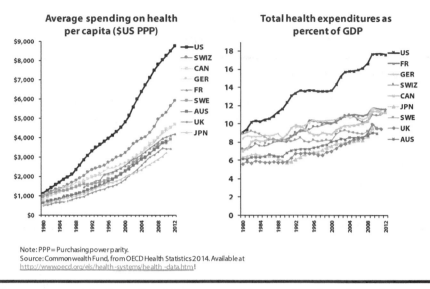

Note: PPP = Purchasing power parity.
Source: Commonwealth Fund, from OECD Health Statistics 2014. Available at
http://www.oecd.org/els/health-systems/health-data.htm!

Figure 2.3   U.S. Spending Higher: Health spending in selected OECD countries, 1980–2012.

Sustaining such inflationary increases is impossible without causing harm to our economy, as health care costs approach 20% of GDP, far in excess of the cost of care in other developed countries (Figure 2.3). Employers, consumers, payers, and government officials are together insisting that health care value should improve [19, 39, 40]. (A more detailed discussion of U.S. health care costs appears in Chapter 6.)

Compared to most industrialized nations, the United States spends a disproportionate percentage of its gross domestic product on health care, while achieving generally poorer outcomes (even after factors like age, racial and ethnic diversity, income, education level, and health insurance status are taken into account) [41, 42]. Factors that appear to drive this higher spending include the higher prevalence of obesity; higher fees for physician services; overuse of diagnostic imaging, procedures, and prescription medications in the United States; poor management of end-of-life care; and proliferation of high-cost medical technology [43–45]. The combination of higher health care spending and poorer outcomes in the

$$\text{Value} = \frac{\text{Quality Outcomes}}{\text{Cost of Episode or condition}}$$

Figure 2.4   Value of care.

United States raises serious questions about the value of the care provided, commonly expressed as quality of care in relation to cost (Figure 2.4). A good understanding of value is important for addressing accountability and the role it plays in improving quality and reducing cost. Throughout this book, value is defined as the quality of health outcomes (e.g., survival and quality of life) that patients achieve relative to the cost of care for the episode or condition described.

Because health care systems have historically not been forced to compete on value, improving the value of health care is challenging. Although we have focused intently on quality for the past 15 years, now in accordance with the Triple Aim, health care providers are challenged to deliver high-quality care and improve population health *while lowering* the cost of care per capita for that population. To date, most of the focus has been on measuring and improving quality of care. Improving population health and reducing per capita costs are somewhat more difficult goals because, in many ways, they lie in opposition to the incentives created by the fee-for-service reimbursement mechanism that dominates the U.S. health care system—which, by basing payments on visits and procedures, rewards providers who *do* more, regardless of the effectiveness or need for that care. Many today are questioning the "more is better" climate prevalent in health care delivery.

The relationship between cost and quality for Medicare beneficiaries is in fact inverse: those states with the highest cost per beneficiary achieve the lowest quality, while those with the lowest cost achieve the highest quality (Figure 2.5).

Further, the Triple Aim advocates improvising the health of populations, some of whom may not encounter the health care system. Hospitals and physicians, paid historically only

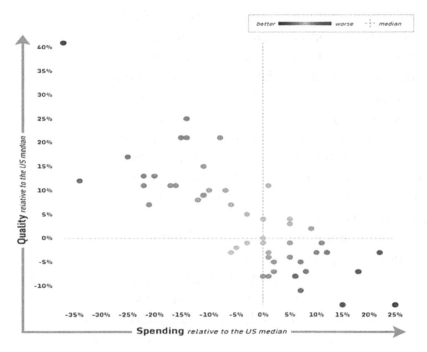

Spending Indicator Source: *Data Year: 2013* – Geographic Variation Public Use File, February 2015 (CMS Office of Information Products and Analytics).

Spending Indicator Notes: Spending estimates exclude prescription drug spending from Medicare Part D and reflect only claims incurred by the age 65+ population with traditional fee-for-service Medicare. Spending estimates are standardized to account for regional differences in wages or input prices, and extra payments that Medicare makes to advance other program goals, such as compensating certain hospitals for the cost of training doctors.

Figure 2.5   Quality and spending relative to the US median for health care.

for transactions, are not paid for care of patients who are not "seen." Clearly, novel payment mechanisms will be needed to achieve the population health mandate of the Triple Aim.

A patient like Mr. B, with multiple chronic uncontrolled conditions being treated in isolation by multiple specialists is likely to require repeated hospitalizations for life-saving interventions as complications develop and progress, which could easily result in more than $50,000 in annual health care costs. These costs of course provide income to his various providers. But what if Mr. B had an established relationship with a PCP, his care was coordinated, his diseases were effectively managed, and he received his preventive health screenings regularly? Would his health outcomes be different? Would he find his health on an improving or at least more stable trajectory? A well-structured, coordinated system of care could certainly reduce redundancies in the care he receives and could potentially halt or slow the progression of his conditions, reducing his need for expensive care (which both Mr. B and any third-party payers would greatly appreciate). However, in the current health care system, his physicians and other providers are not reimbursed for the time spent on that coordination, and excessive time spent on those activities would actually lower their incomes.

ACO models that provide the infrastructure and financial incentives (i.e., shared savings, bundled payments, pay for performance, and capitation) to facilitate improved patient outcomes through collaboration across the care continuum are one of the innovations in health care organizations in the United States that many industry leaders hope will facilitate the transformation needed to efficiently and effectively manage care for the growing number of patients with complex conditions like Mr. B [46, 47]. These incentives are intended to mitigate the loss of income that will result from reduced need for specialist visits, procedures, and hospitalization with better disease management, through a combination of shared savings and replacement patient volume. For example, the ACO, by attracting contracts and covered lives, can encourage in-network referrals and help backfill the excess capacity created by reducing unnecessary utilization. To accomplish this, ACOs require a structure that is "bottom heavy," with large numbers of PCPs (who typically serve as the point from which patients' care is coordinated) and who feed into a relatively small number of physicians in each relevant specialty. Supporting this structure may require a fundamental shift in the U.S. physician workforce development. It will require finding ways to attract and reward more physicians to comprehensive primary care careers rather than the specialties that offer greater financial reward, more prestige, and more flexible schedules. It may also necessitate transforming primary care itself into teams of highly regarded "comprehensivists" supported by greater use of nurse practitioners, physician assistants, nurses, and expanded care teams.

Accountability for Clinical Integration

"I did my part." Many of us have heard physicians and others make such statements in the care of complex patients, even though the overall patient outcome was poor. For example, a successful atrial fibrillation ablation may be very good, but it will seem a poor outcome to a patient who suffers a stroke a week after the procedure. While everyone values the best skill and expertise, delivery of that skilled care is often only as effective as what happens before and after that episode or procedure. Certainly, patients are "whole" even when we mostly treat their "parts."

The emergence of the hospitalist movement has highlighted the need for connecting or integrating care across the continuum of care from community to hospital and back. Multiple providers are often involved in those hospitalization episodes, sometimes resulting in redundancy, conflicting advice, and dropped hand-offs. Today, nurses working in care transitions between hospital discharge and community care report that most patients misunderstand medication instructions (BSWQA nurse care managers, personal communication). Our usual care systems often have deficiencies surrounding transitions and complex care.

In traditional care, the patient or a caregiver may have to serve as a navigator between specialists and sites of care. Fortunate indeed is the frail, widowed elderly man whose loyal daughter accompanies him to multiple specialist visits, carrying personal health records in a three-ring binder. She knows the system doesn't naturally integrate, so she is the self-appointed integrator for her father.

In an accountable system, this could all change. The medical record could be electronically available at all sites.

The care would be evidence based and heavily driven by protocols and care paths. The patient would have a personal comprehensivist PCP and a PCMH to help guide, reconcile, and translate the complexity of multiple practitioners. His wishes and preferences would all be respected, including preemptive discussion of end-of-life preferences. Non-value-adding costly tests and procedures would be avoided. And all of those parties involved in his case would hold themselves *accountable* for communicating and coordinating their expertise in his interest.

Accountable by Whom and to Whom?

As described earlier in this chapter, being *accountable* means having the obligation to make all decisions in the interest of quality and cost-effectiveness for patients and to address patient wishes regarding decisions and actions [21, 48]. In the ACO model, physicians, hospitals, and other providers hold themselves responsible for achieving these aims illustrated by transparent performance measures that reflect the goals of better overall health of patients through higher-quality care and lower costs. These reports will document whether (or not) the ACO has indeed improved performance across the domains of patient experience, care coordination, patient safety, and preventive care, with particular attention to at-risk populations [49]. The governance structure of an ACO that ensures accountability generally includes both administrative and clinical managers, who coordinate efforts to deliver improved care at a lower cost. Administrative leaders must oversee the ACO's interaction with payers, the coordination of the ACO operations with ACO participants and partners, the production and dissemination of quality and financial data, and the administration of policies for reward distribution. Clinical leadership roles in an ACO generally focus on ensuring that the best care is provided in the most economical setting for ACO patients through establishment of care coordination guidelines, review and dissemination of best practice information, and practice improvement (including identification of providers with outlier practice patterns, along with strategies for their clinical improvement) [50].

Even drug manufacturers and device makers are challenged to be accountable through the ACO structure. For example, as ACOs pursue ways to deliver high-quality care at the lowest cost, most are asking their members to increase generic medication prescribing rates and are seeking to purchase medical devices that have the best track records with respect to lowering hospital readmission rates and preventing hospital-acquired complications. Additionally, ACO purchasing decisions are less likely to rely on individual physician preference and are more likely to depend on group purchasing decisions, incentivizing more widespread accountability for manufacturers and device makers to demonstrate their products' superior effectiveness and cost [51].

Physicians, hospitals, providers, and suppliers are all held accountable *by* ACOs; they are accountable for both individual patients and specific patient populations (i.e., a defined group of the organization's patients; see Chapter 5) [52]. While health care providers have always been accountable to individual patients, the concept of accountability to patient populations is relatively new. Under a fee-for-service, payment-for-volume health care model, providers are reimbursed for specific patient transactions or care experiences. A fee-for-value model, in contrast, emphasizes and rewards the ACO's role in maintaining and enhancing the health of attributed patients over time, whether seen in care settings or not. An ACO may still rely on fee-for-service-based billing methods as providers experiment with different payment models, but in most cases, providers ultimately accept some financial risk for their accountable care patient population [53]. Successful management of population health requires the adoption and implementation of a variety of initiatives, including health management programs (e.g., wellness visits), disease management programs,

transparent communication of outcomes to payers, to employers, and to patients, robust data infrastructure for measuring
and reporting outcomes, financial consequences for suboptimal performance, and committed leadership [46, 54, 55].

Accountable Care Structures

The ACA sanctioned ACOs in 2010, authorizing the Centers for
Medicare and Medicaid Services (CMS) MSSP under Section
3022 and the Pioneer ACO models, as well as establishment of
the Center for Medicare and Medicaid Innovation, to test new
payment models [14]. The intent of both these programs was
for participating organizations to try to lower Medicare costs
while meeting stringent quality standards, with the incentive to
do so being receipt of a portion of the resultant savings. While
the ACA did not formally address the formation of private or
commercial ACOs, these have also proliferated in its wake: in
2014, there were at least 626 ACOs across the United States,
including 329 with government contracts, 210 with commercial contracts, 74 with both, and 13 that had not announced or
finalized the nature of their contracts [15, 50]. These organizations have brought physicians, hospitals, and others together
to hold themselves contractually accountable for improving
quality of care, lowering costs, and better integrating and
coordinating care for the patients served. Like various other
payment reforms (e.g., value-based purchasing and bundled
payments) being implemented or tested in the U.S. health care
system, ACOs are part of the movement attempting to transition from paying for volume to paying for value. Although
many ACOs are struggling to lower cost, the successful ACOs
have lowered cost, improved quality, and rewarded participants with some financial rewards [49, 56, 57]. Performance
for participating physicians and hospital members is measured
and distributed across the ACO, and all of the participants are
asked to be *accountable* for improvement.

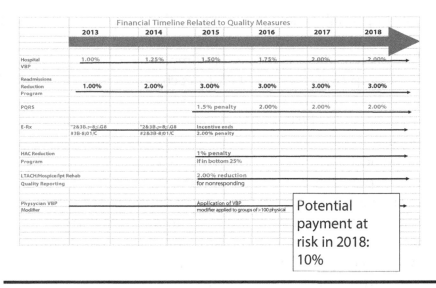

Figure 2.6 Medicare payment at risk under CMS quality-based payment reform initiatives.

Most leaders in the ACO environment recognize that there is a long road ahead to achieve the levels of accountability required to truly reform our system and bring the best value possible to our patients [58, 59]. CMS is leading the way in shifting to value-based payment, announcing in 2015 increasing percentages of payments tied to value-based care (Figure 2.6). At the 2015 Healthcare Leadership Council on Value and Innovation, a coalition of providers, payers, patients, and regulators agreed that payment reform will become essential to achieving the best value. Health care delivery involves many complex cultures and subcultures, making change difficult. Traditional care processes and payment models may have to be replaced or redesigned for the new models of care to function. Old habits may need to yield and bend so superior outcomes can be achieved. Evidence-based standardization will challenge both individual and organizational autonomy. Aspects of these changes are likely to be disruptive to every health care stakeholder—patient, provider, payer, and supplier— and *accountability* will be required on both individual and corporate levels. Can our systems reform themselves?

Mr. B is unlikely to be considering the complexities of reforming the health care system. From his point of view, it likely seems that the solution is simple: his doctors and other care providers should talk to each other, pool their information, and come up with a strategy that can improve and maintain his health in a cost-efficient manner. The red tape and complexity that thwart his attempts to receive the care he needs are as likely to adversely affect him as any of his current health problems—a perception that is sadly accurate should it prevent him from receiving the coordinated disease management he needs from an *accountable* care system and providers. There is little Mr. B can do, other than stay informed about his health conditions and try to be an active participant in his care. Only health care leaders are in a position to redesign the system and connect the siloed aspects of medical care to create a coordinated system that can effectively and efficiently change his outcomes. Do we not owe it to Mr. B to do so?

Chapter 3

Structure and Organization: Putting an Accountable Care Organization Together

Main Points for Chapter

This chapter includes a discussion of:

- How an accountable care organization is structured and governed
- Legal requirements, considerations, and implications for accountable care organizations
- The importance of data, care coordination, and transitions in care in an accountable care world
- How health care access and primary care drive accountability

Three physician leaders of a large, independent, 60-person radiology group had requested a meeting with the BSWQA leadership. They were contemplating joining the ACO but had some questions. One was, "Why should we join the ACO? Isn't the organization going to reduce the use of imaging?" As president of BSWQA, my reply was, "Do you think that in the near future, health care reform will result in a reduction of radiologic imaging per 1,000 patients whether you join or not?"

They nodded in agreement.

I then asked if I could step out of my executive role in BSWQA and pretend to give practice advice. "If I were your manager and all the physicians wanted to read the same volume of films and images, given the coming utilization reductions and an avoidance of waste in the reform era, I would suggest that you have too many radiologists and should shrink your group to 50. Alternatively, if the ACO is successful and we bring a better value to the market, we should gain thousands of lives, and perhaps backfill your capacity."

They joined the ACO.

Structure of Accountable Care Organizations

Organizational Models for Accountable Care Organizations

The definition of and requirements for Medicare ACOs established in the ACA give organizations broad latitude in determining their organizational structure. Outside the Medicare context, there can be even greater flexibility: for example, Texas passed legislation in 2011 authorizing the creation of "health care collaborations" by physicians, hospitals, and other health care providers; this legislation was intended to provide greater flexibility around the quality measures and payment methods used [60]. This intentional latitude enables providers to structure their ACOs according to what resources they already have, what local partners are interested in forming an ACO, and what is most needed in their local community. As a result, there is substantial variation both in how ACOs are organized and in how categories of ACOs are described or classified. These generally revolve around who the sponsoring entities [61], owners [62], and leaders [63] are, but no well-defined classification system has been agreed upon. The most comprehensive classification system takes into account the ACO's number of full-time member physicians and the percentage of these who are PCPs, types of included provider organizations or services offered, ownership by an integrated delivery system, institutional leadership model, performance management system for accountability, and prior experience with non-fee-for-service payment mechanisms [64]. Based on these measures, three "clusters" of ACOs have been identified. These are outlined in Table 3.1.

BSWQA was built on the foundations of clinical integration that had been established within the BHCS (which included acute, specialty, and post–acute care facilities) and HTPN. At its current network size of almost 4,000 physicians, BSWQA falls into the category of a very large integrated delivery system.

Qualities of Physician-Hospital-Led versus Physician-Led Accountable Care Organizations

In the first couple of years of the ACO movement, hospital systems were the predominant sponsoring entities and leaders [61], but by 2013 ACOs led by physician groups or jointly led by hospitals and physician groups accounted for almost 75% of all ACOs [63]. These models each offer different challenges and benefits.

Table 3.1 Classification of Accountable Care Organizations

Large integrated delivery system ACOs	■ Average size: 566 full-time clinicians
	■ 40% report being physician led
	■ Relatively low percentage of PCPs (42.5%)
	■ Broad scope of services across the continuum of care
	■ Relatively experienced with alternative reimbursement mechanisms
	■ Score low on the use of performance measurement and accountability mechanisms
	■ Account for 40% of ACOs
Smaller physician-led ACOs	■ Average size: 181 full-time clinicians
	■ 91% report being physician led
	■ High percentage of PCPs (68.8%)
	■ Narrow scope of services offered
	■ Least experience with alternative reimbursement mechanisms
	■ Score highest on use of performance measurement and accountability mechanisms
	■ Account for 34% of ACOs
Hybrid ACOs	■ Average size: 42 full-time clinicians
	■ 21% report being physician led
	■ The remainder tended to be hospital, coalition, or state, region, or county led
	■ Relatively high percentage of PCPs (58.5%)
	■ Broad scope of services offered
	■ Relatively experienced with alternative reimbursement mechanisms
	■ Score lowest on use of performance measurement and accountability mechanisms
	■ Account for 28% of ACOs

Source: Shortell, S.M., et al., *Health Serv Res*, 2014; 49(6): 1883–99.

For physician-led ACOs, challenges include the need to establish clinical, administrative, and fiscal cooperation with a variety of other providers—relationships that many physicians practicing in small or solo practices may have little experience with initiating or maintaining [65]. Without the infrastructure and resources of a larger organization, such as a hospital or integrated delivery system, for example, they might also struggle with the necessary capital investment (including funding for HIT), assumption of financial risk, and allocation and distribution of gains or losses [65]. On the other hand, they are well positioned to improve the prevention and management of chronic diseases, and prevent the need for expensive ED visits or hospital admissions—without having a hospital's conflicting concern of how preventing admissions will affect the bottom line. While the majority of physicians remain unenthusiastic about eliminating the fee-for-service payment model for their services [66], their reimbursement is relatively easy to transition from volume to value payments without necessitating substantial loss in revenue. In contrast, when an ACO is successful in reducing its population's health care resource utilization, the only way for a hospital to sustain its former level of revenue is to increase its market share—for which it must compete with other hospitals facing a similar ultimatum. Physicians in procedure-based specialties as in our opening story (e.g., radiologists) are in a situation similar to that of hospitals in the ACO context, facing reduced revenue as accountable care both reduces unnecessary utilization and, by improving overall health, reduces the need for utilization of some specialty services.

The 2012–2013 survey of ACOs shows that physician-led ACOs have found ways to overcome some but not all of these challenges: while they have management and HIT capabilities similar to those of ACOs with other leadership structures, they are less likely to include a hospital or provide emergency, rehabilitation, behavioral health, skilled nursing, pediatric, palliative or hospice, home health, or pharmacy services, suggesting they may have difficulty improving coordination and transitions of complex care between providers and settings [63].

Introducing hospital leadership to an ACO triggers a different set of considerations. Hospitals can provide many of the administrative, financial, and coordinating resources needed for success, and their leaders may have more experience with establishing the types of collaborative arrangements an ACO is likely to need for success. In addition, incorporating hospitals into an ACO offers more opportunities to improve quality and efficiency of care, both because it involves and aligns more of the people whose decisions influence care and costs and because it facilitates work around care transitions in a setting that is one of the highest cost drivers in health care. However, participation and leadership in an ACO require a hospital to make some fundamental changes that disrupt the fee-for-service business model—especially if payers do not alter their payment mechanisms simultaneously. Historically, hospitals have focused on procedures and severely ill patients, often profitably. Success in the ACO context, however, will decrease the per capita demand for admissions and procedures in the population the ACO serves, straining the resources of providers who rely on those to generate revenue. As such, not all hospitals may be able to make the required shift to a more outpatient-focused, population-based, coordinated care model, forgoing some short-term profits from procedures and admissions in favor of long-term savings [65]. Hospitals and health care systems are also more likely to have established relationships with other providers within the continuum of care that may influence how or how much the ACO can accountably change the quality and cost of care provided. For example, BSWQA encountered this in the form of joint ventures with ambulatory surgery centers and imaging services in the BSWH North Texas division. Such entities can be important revenue sources for a health care system but may not offer the lowest cost in the local market and are volume-oriented. The preexisting relationship, which incorporates these providers into the ACO without their having to demonstrate their ability to meet cost and quality standards set by the ACO, coupled with the health care system's dependence on the revenue they generate, can reduce the ACO's opportunities for reducing costs of care by contracting for these services with lower-cost providers. Instead, value has to be improved by focusing on eliminating overuse and, in the long term, working with the joint venture partners, holding them *accountable* to reduce their costs.

ACOs that arc jointly lcd by hospitals and physician groups have taken different approaches to balancing the potentially conflicting interests and to ensuring the focus remains on the ACO's overall mission of improving population health while decreasing health care costs. Advocate Physician Partners in Illinois, for example, formed its ACO from a clinically integrated joint venture between Advocate Health Care (a not-for-profit health care system with ten hospital campuses) and the partnership physicians associated with each of its hospitals through a local physician-hospital organization (PHO). It created two membership classes with equal numbers of governance votes: one for the health care system and one for the PHOs. For any measure to pass, a majority of votes within each of these classes is required. Furthermore, many of the health care system's governance seats are occupied by employed physicians rather than administrators, creating a physician super majority and a structure within which physicians and hospitals can work on improving care with common quality and cost-effectiveness goals [67].

Building on Existing Infrastructure

BSWQA was initially established on the foundations of the integration between the multihospital not-for profit BHCS and its affiliated medical group practice HTPN, with more than 300 National Committee for Quality Assurance (NCQA) Level 3 PCMH–certified PCPs. This enabled BSWQA to largely avoid

many of the growing pains related to integration that many
ACOs experience, such as inadequate integration of enter-
prise systems, slow uptake of EHRs in physician practices, and
poor communication among ambulatory care, in-patient, and
post–acute care [68]. HTPN had already implemented a common EHR across its practices, was working on transforming its
primary care practices into accredited PCMHs (standardizing
many of the elements essential to population health management across the network), and was establishing an ambulatory
care coordination department to target patient care advocacy,
hospital discharge transition and follow-up, preventive services, and disease management [69]. Meanwhile, BHCS was
nearing completion on the rollout of a uniform EHR and
computerized physician order entry system across its hospitals.
Both BHCS and HTPN also had a decade of experience with
various forms of performance measurement and reporting,
including pay-for-performance programs that tie portions
of hospital leaders' and physicians' reimbursement to this
performance [69–71], and had a long history of collaborating
on quality improvement initiatives, investing in each other's
infrastructure and participating in each other's governance
structures [69].

While BSWQA has not divided its 21 governance seats
between health care system and physician group representatives in a formal manner like Advocate Physician Partners,
its board of managers is structured to ensure adequate
representation of stakeholders by including physicians
(selected from multiple medical staff communities to represent
all parts of the BSWH system as well as HTPN), executives,
and members of the community. As BSWQA has expanded,
adding independent physician members and, with the 2013
merger between BHCS and SWH, the SWH hospitals and the
employed physicians within SWH clinics, additional leaders
representing these groups have been brought onto the board
of managers [72].

Network Building

To be fully effective, an ACO needs to develop a right-sized, appropriately distributed network of physicians, other providers of care, social services, hospitals, and post–acute care providers to cover the full continuum of health care and wellness needs for the population for which it is accountable [73]. Since that population can change over time as the ACO contracts with different payers and employers, the network must be dynamic to some degree, with frequent checks of its adequacy to identify any gaps that may have developed.

The PCPs within the network form the backbone of the ACO. This is because primary care is typically the main point of contact with the ACO (and with clinical care in general) for individuals within the population for which the ACO is accountable, as well as the setting through which the majority of population health management activities and chronic disease management occur [74]. Additionally, because the ACO includes hospitals and specialist physicians, the PCP members are a critical source of referrals for those providers. As population health management is coupled with initiatives to identify and eliminate overuse of health care resources, increasing numbers of PCPs referring patients to them will be needed. As such, a significant long-term challenge, not just for BSWQA but for the broader goal of improving population health and reducing health care expenditures, is the shortage of PCPs in the United States [75].

In its northern region, BSWQA started with a strong base of primary care practices through HTPN, which has more than 325 PCPs practicing at more than 90 locations in and around the Dallas–Fort Worth metroplex. However, as BSWQA started acquiring more covered lives through its contracts with different payers and benefit plans, it needed to recruit more independent physician practices. This is particularly true in the western part of Fort Worth, where HTPN does not have as strong a presence as in Dallas.

With the 2013 merger with SWH, BSWQA expanded its reach to the central Texas region. Again, it acquired a comprehensive network of physicians in the area when SWH clinics (with more than 1,100 employed physicians) joined BSWQA with a good primary care base and full complement of specialists.

In developing its network, BSWQA has had two phases. The first of these involved widespread education and engagement of the physician community in the targeted area on the topic of ACOs in general and participation in BSWQA in particular. Important forums for this message included holding regional POD (i.e., groups of physicians organized by region) meetings and attending local practice meetings, as well as extensive use of a robust interactive member website. From a recruitment perspective, good candidates included physicians with experience with risk-based contracts, and large independent practice associations or health care systems. Physicians experienced with risk-based contracts generally understand the mission of the ACO intuitively and are able to serve as local leaders or champions, encouraging their less experienced colleagues to join and be effective participants in the ACO. These physician leaders are more likely to be accustomed to working within a centralized structure and to appreciate the benefits of coordination and standardization it facilitates. BSWQA's alignment with BSWH presented a challenge in recruiting large independent practice associations because many of them either are aligned with one of the other large health care systems in the region, and so are reluctant to "join the competition," or have deliberately remained independent of *all* the health care systems because they value their autonomy over the efficiencies alignment can provide. BSWQA elected to not require exclusivity in members; they were free to join other ACOs as well.

The second phase of network maturation is very operationally focused: looking at the anticipated BSWQA contractual growth in covered lives and then comparing the distribution of the existing network together with payer data to determine exactly what types of service need to be added in geographic sub-regions. In areas where BSWQA does not yet have any covered lives, it assumes that it will be accountable for at least one life in each zip code and makes the determination of what services would be needed to provide average coverage for each of those lives. As covered lives are acquired, this analysis reverses: looking at where the members of the population for which BSWQA is accountable reside, does the network provide adequate access for every covered life?

BSWQA's primary care adequacy analysis is based on a ten-mile geo-access requirement for internal medicine, family medicine, and pediatric physicians. It considers adequacy from the perspective of both meeting the state insurance agency standards [76] and marketability to individuals and employers. This latter consideration takes into account such factors as driving ten miles to see a physician in a rural versus an urban area, the inclusion in an employee population of commuters for whom access near home is more important than access near the employer, and the fact that access requires not merely physicians in the right area but also physicians with available capacity.

With only 18% of the BSWQA network being PCPs, most of BSWQA's network building efforts now focus on primary care capacity, with specialists tending to follow through either their connections to the recruited PCPs or affiliations with a BSWQA member hospital. An additional focus on adequate ob-gyn membership has also been identified. All the payers with whom BSWQA contracts test the network's adequacy every six months, either by testing the total and available capacity of the BSWQA physicians against their real population of enrollees in the region or by using geo-access analysis. A map depicting federally designated health professional shortages for primary care in the state of Texas appears in Figure 3.1.

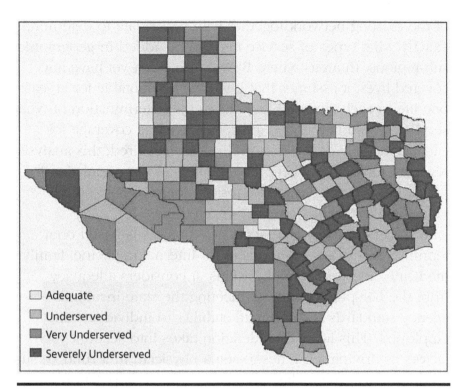

Figure 3.1 Health professional shortages for primary care in Texas. (From *Texas Tribune*, Interactive: mapping access to health care in Texas, May 8, 2012, http://www.texastribune.org/library/data/texas-shortage-health-care-providers/?%20utm_source=texastribune. org&utm_medium=alerts&utm_campaign=News%20Alert:%20 Subscriptions.)

Another area in which BSWQA has focused its network-building efforts is in post–acute care—a basic requirement for population management, particularly in senior care. Post–acute care is often poorly integrated with both physician and hospital care. It is also a very high-cost area within the care continuum [78] and has a history of fraud and abuse [79], making high-quality, *accountable*, post–acute care providers' acceptance for membership critical to BSWQA's long-term success in improving the quality and cost-effectiveness of care for its population. Approximately 30 skilled nursing facilities, ten home health agencies, and three rehabilitation centers have been invited to join BSWQA and have accepted. To promote alignment and integration with the ambulatory and acute care providers within BSWQA, the medical directors of participating post–acute care providers are required to be BSWQA members. Coordination and integration of patient care is also facilitated through regular visits by nurse care managers from the BSWQA care coordination department to members of the ACO's contract population receiving post–acute care in those facilities. Performance metrics on which post–acute care providers report data to BSWQA include avoidable hospital readmissions, completion rates of advance directives, falls, and the continuation of care paths initiated during a hospitalization. These metrics are compared and transparent on the secure website.

Physicians within the Accountable Care Organization

Physicians joining BSWQA, regardless of whether they either fall within the BSWH-employed physician groups or are in independent practice, must meet certain requirements and sign a participation agreement committing their efforts to be personally *accountable* for fulfilling BSWQA's mission of improving quality, clinically integrating, and reducing the overall cost of care for the populations it serves (see Chapter 4 for a more detailed description of these requirements). This and the performance standards required to qualify for shared savings are the principal mechanisms through which physicians are organized within BSWQA. They commit to submitting data for measurement of both clinical and cost-effective performance and to remediation of performance that is inadequate.

Employed Physicians versus Independent Physicians

The relative attributes of the hospital-employed versus independent physician models have been debated, particularly around the questions of quality and productivity [80]. In an

ACO structured like BSWQA, it may ultimately make little difference since employed and independent physicians must meet the same requirements, are held to the same clinical and cost standards, receive the same performance reports, and are eligible for the same rewards. To date, within BSWQA, the employed and independent physicians have raised similar questions about the performance data being reported and have expressed similar opinions about how ACOs need to be physician driven. Where this can make a difference is in recruitment (since physicians in employed groups can be told they have to either join the ACO or find other employment), in familiarity with the process of receiving performance reports, in working within the structures of a larger organization, and in the practice resources they have available to them to meet the requirements for participation and the quality performance standards.

HTPN has been tracking and reporting quality performance measures for its physicians since the 1990s [71]. These physicians are accustomed to seeing these objective measures not merely of their own performance but of their transparent performance relative to that of their peers, and they value that data as a tool to help ensure they deliver the evidence-based care their patients need. They have overcome the initial reaction of resistance and distrust of the data. Skeptical reactions can be expected from physicians recruited in BSWQA from other practice settings where they have not had access to the infrastructure needed to support this type of quality measurement, nor any oversight requiring it. BSWQA is applying the lessons learned from the HTPN experience in how to overcome the negative reactions to performance reporting, for example, by appointing physician champions who can meet one-on-one with the member physicians to explain both how the reports are generated and how they can help improve practice. Also helpful is the detailed level of reporting that is now possible because the reports generated enable the data to be viewed at the practice, physician, and patient levels, the last of which enables physicians to verify the reports against their own clinical records.

Physicians who entered BSWQA through SWH clinics likewise have extensive experience with organizational initiatives aimed at improving quality and efficiency that independent physicians may be encountering for the first time within BSWQA. For example, SWH clinics have focused extensively on improving access to primary care, not only by recruiting PCPs but also by instituting team-based care and adding advanced practitioners to primary care practices. This is an approach likely to become more and more necessary as ACOs advance their population health management services, but such "sharing" of clinical responsibilities takes time for physicians to become acclimated [81]. SWH clinics have also been operated for years as tightly integrated primary-specialty multidisciplinary units; BSWQA has identified "best practices" from these integrated models and is seeking to spread them throughout its wide network.

Another area in which independent and employed physicians might have very different experiences in an ACO is in the resources available to them to meet the criteria for membership or to receive shared savings. While ACOs can provide resources or support to independent physicians for some items—for example, a financial subsidy for acquiring an EHR [82, 83] and provision of care coordination services for those patients insured through plans that have contracted with BSWQA—their ability to do so in other areas is limited. For example, one of the 2015 criteria for PCPs within BSWQA to receive a portion of any shared savings is that their practice had, at a minimum, submitted an application to the NCQA for recognition as a PCMH. When HTPN practices engaged in this process in 2011 and 2012, and now as they submit applications for renewal, HTPN was able to create a group within its corporate structure to lead this work, providing tools to help practices meet the NCQA standards as well as writing and submitting the actual applications. For the independent practices,

BSWQA is legally limited to providing examples of how successful applicants have met the standards and advising the practices about the application process as consultants.

A final important area in which independent physicians' relationship with or functioning within an ACO may be at least temporarily different is the ability to access EHR data for patients in the ACO's population as they move between points of care. All BSWH-employed physician practices have implemented a common EHR, enabling any employed physician treating a patient to access and add to the patient's record directly in the EHR at the point of care anywhere he or she has a secure Internet connection. Similar access is not available to independent physicians (who may have implemented different, or even incompatible EHRs). Thus, when a patient within the BSWQA accountable population whose PCMH is with one of the independent BSWQA PCPs is referred to an HTPN-affiliated specialist within BSWQA or is admitted to a BSWH hospital and is treated by a hospitalist physician, the patient's EHR is not accessible at the point of care. The same holds true when the PCP in the scenario is part of HTPN but the hospitalist is not. Within the 2,200 independent physician practices, over 70 different brands of EHRs were found. To solve this problem, BSWQA is implementing an interoperable health information exchange (HIE), which will connect the disparate EHR systems by appearing on both systems as an "agent" that produces an aggregate record for the patient. The HIE will enable not only promote the connection of the disparate EHR systems within BSWQA, but also the integration of BSWQA's data analytics systems. This technology will allow simultaneous reporting of a patient's medical history, demographics, risk status, cost information, and other data relevant to population health management, enabling better-informed shared decision making between patients and physicians at the point of care [84]. The clinical integration benefits of this HIE are already being realized.

Disruptive Effect of Volume to Value

> There are two basic approaches to developing health
> policies. The first, which is cautious and careful
> (a small idea and a small intervention or even a
> big idea and a small intervention), is more likely
> to be tested and implemented because institutions
> and professionals will not be threatened by the
> magnitude of the change....
>
> The second approach is disruptive and daring
> (big idea and big intervention). It can adequately
> test a concept, but the concept may be dismissed
> as infeasible. [85]

Disruptive innovations are risky—most of them fail—so
they are less likely to receive research funding or be implemented within the health care system [85]. The shift from vol-
ume- to value-based payment in health care (see Chapter 6
for more details), including the associated formation of ACOs,
is fundamentally a disruptive change. To date, however,
its implementation has been relatively small. Even health
care providers that have taken the more dramatic plunge
into the world of risk-based contracting by participating in
the Pioneer ACO demonstration project report that more
than 80% of their patients continue to be cared for under
a fee-for-service model [86]. This duality of practice draws
focus and momentum away from the cost reduction, disease
prevention, and population health that value-based payment
is intended to motivate. How can physicians, hospitals, and
others deal with this duality of patient types and reimbursement methods? For instance, an ACO patient may have clinical
access to ambulatory care coordinators, who are funded by
value-based payments, whereas a fee-for-service patient may
not have that resource. Because of the transactional nature of
fee-for-service payments, those funds are usually nonexistent.
Further, clinicians are asked in value-based ACO contracts to

avoid unnecessary costs, preventable admissions, and avoidable ED visits. In fee-for-service payment models, those events are actually reimbursable and rarely scrutinized. Physician and hospital leaders are increasingly finding that the skill in managing two different types of payment is a form of ambidexterity. We have been experts in managing the right-handedness of fee-for-service reimbursements. Today we are learning to throw skillfully with the left-handed value-based payment environment and to be *accountable* for the results. This may be changing, however: in early 2015, the Department of Health and Human Services announced that it aims to have 30% of payments for traditional Medicare benefits tied to alternative payment models such as ACOs by the end of 2016, and 50% by the end of 2018. On the hospital side, the goals are even more ambitious: moving from the 20% of Medicare payments for traditional beneficiaries currently made through alternative payment models to 85% being made through quality- or value-based programs such as the Hospital Value-Based Purchasing, Hospital Readmissions Reduction Program, bundled payments by the end of 2016, and 90% alternative payments by the end of 2018 [87]. Assuming other payers follow suit, this degree of implementation on this aggressive timeline may provide the level of disruption needed to effect the changes necessary to halt and reverse rising U.S. health care costs. ACOs, by providing structures within which the transition can occur and by motivating early change among participating providers *despite* ongoing contradictory incentives created by the fee-for-service reimbursement that still dominates the industry, can cushion the landing as the value-based payment model gains momentum and critical mass. Figure 3.2 displays a hypothetical example of how, over time, the proportion of value-based payments relative to volume-based payments can increase. The rising percentage of value-based payments drives an enhanced focus on value throughout the health care system. However, as value-based payments increase, the effect on practice patterns is likely to affect all patient types.

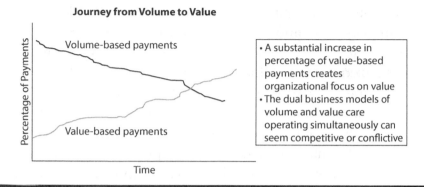

Journey from Volume to Value

- Volume-based payments
- Value-based payments

Percentage of Payments

Time

- A substantial increase in percentage of value-based payments creates organizational focus on value
- The dual business models of volume and value care operating simultaneously can seem competitive or conflictive

Figure 3.2   Journey from volume to value.

In terms of health care structures, the disruptive effect of the movement toward value-based payments can be seen at all levels of the health care system. At the macro level, providers have been seeking safety in numbers—with hospitals consolidating into large multihospital health care systems and physician practices merging—and in vertical integration, with physicians increasingly working in practices owned by or aligned with a hospital or health care system [88, 89]. Motivations behind these changes in organizational structure include the need to make the capital investments (particularly in HIT and data infrastructure) necessary to succeed in many alternative payment models, greater bargaining power to negotiate contracts with health plans, acquisition of the infrastructure and capabilities needed for the prevention and care coordination focus of value-based payment models, and the efficiencies and economies of scale [89, 90]. But at the micro level, practice patterns must change.

Disruptions are occurring within individual hospitals and physician practices as they seek to adapt to the new model. A notable example is the increased adoption of team approaches to care management—particularly in primary care settings—with practices finding ways within the PCMH and shared savings models to fund advanced practice providers and care manager or care coordinator positions. Care coordinators concentrate on patient management between

office visits and identification of gaps in recommended disease management and preventive services, freeing physician
time during office visits for clinical care [89]. BSWQA provides
a centralized care coordination resource (described below)
and designed it specifically to generate sufficient income in
the current fee-for-service-dominated environment to cover
the currently unreimbursed time spent reviewing patient
records and contacting patients via telephone to coordinate
needed care, improve preventive services, and support disease
management. These currently unreimbursed services will be
critical to success as greater proportions of the primary care
practices' income comes through value-based payment mechanisms. For example, care coordinators may set up primary care
appointments for wellness visits or post–hospital discharge
follow-up visits that might otherwise slip through the cracks.
Such visits represent lost revenue as well as missed opportunities for prevention and disease management activities that
reduce risk for adverse outcomes. Another "disruption" occurring at the provider level is the need to offer patients expanded
access to after-hours care (including email, telephone, and web
portal communication with the physician practice, as well as
alternative care site options like retail clinics and urgent care
centers)—discussed in detail in Chapter 4.

Finally, value-based payment models seek to change how
physicians think about and act in their clinical practices. The
ambidexterity required in transition necessitates resources,
training, and data. Rather than representing each patient as a
single case with an isolated problem, the value-based payment
models want clinicians also to coordinate individual patients'
care across providers. This coordination is facilitated by such
tools as universal patient records, so that all physicians treating a patient seeing multiple specialists have access to results
from all the tests run, procedures performed and medications
prescribed, to avoid duplication and conflicting interventions,
and to consider the care they provide from the perspective
of their entire patient population (facilitated by performance

measurement reports). Key to both of these changes are data—how they are collected and used to drive practice. This is discussed in detail in Chapter 5.

While the fee-for-service payment model continues to dominate the market, organizations like BSWQA must constantly remind their members—both physicians and hospitals—that while disruption of the traditional structures and practices may be uncomfortable in the short term, there are long-term benefits to be reaped through preparedness for the widespread adoption of value-based payment mechanisms. Providers who have not developed the competencies and relationships necessary to responsibly manage the financial risk for the care of most, if not all, of their patients may face a sharp, unpleasant awakening. On a personal level, *accountable* practice changes will be required to successfully move into the new world of value-based payment.

Interactions with Health Plans

Insurers can be involved in ACOs in multiple ways, including contracting for covered lives with an ACO, being the sponsoring entity that organizes providers into an ACO and assumes the risk of providing accountable care, or partnering with a provider organization to create an ACO in which stakeholders both assume some of the risk and provide services aimed at improving population health and decreasing overall costs [61]. Particularly large insurer organizations have played instrumental roles in ACO development, especially through investments in competencies to enable care coordination and through promotion and sponsoring of risk-based arrangements with both small and large provider organizations [61].

BSWQA contracts with multiple insurers but, because of the BHCS-SWH merger, has a unique relationship with the provider-owned Scott & White Health Plan that offers a strong basis for a fully integrated delivery network. This relationship enables coordination of efforts and maximizes use of each organization's strengths. Because of the common ownership, both organizations stand to benefit when total costs of care are reduced, and since ED visits and hospital stays are some of the greatest cost drivers in health care, both entities are interested in preventing these. Rather than duplicating efforts and resources, however, BSWQA and the Scott & White Health Plan have identified two groups of patients at high risk for these events and are each focusing on one. The first group are patients with multiple chronic conditions, which BSWQA, with its strong focus on primary care and population health management, is targeting for care coordination and case management to prevent disease progression, adverse drug events, and other factors that can precipitate the need for acute care. The other group is multiple trauma patients, which the Scott & White Health Plan is targeting for care coordination at transitions between care settings, and to ensure appropriate post–acute care to reduce risk of unplanned readmissions during what may be a long and complex recovery.

Other areas where BSWQA and the Scott & White Health Plan are working to coordinate their efforts and avoid duplication for the contract population include the identification and management of patients in the "rising risk" category for chronic diseases and the wellness and biometric screening programs, which include such services as health coaching and linkage of the insured patient with the provider network (including, for new health plan enrollees, the offer of a scheduled appointment with a PCP upon enrollment).

BSWQA and the Scott & White Health Plan also intersect at the point of building marketable insurance products. BSWQA will contribute a network of providers across the care continuum, assuring, through the standards it sets as requirements for membership and criteria that must be met to receive shared savings, that these providers offer high-quality care at reasonable costs. Simultaneously, the Scott & White Health Plan will use its experience, data, and resources to design, market, and manage insurance products built around this network. These products could include, for example, tailored network plans that can be offered at lower cost, as well as tiered plans that offer broader consumer choice of provider but incorporate strong incentives steering consumers toward the BSWQA network. BSWQA has been the preferred network for BSWH–North Texas employees since 2012 and used a third party administrator carrier prior to the merger. As a self-insured employer, BSWH offered plan design alternatives to employees to encourage in-network utilization. For example, in 2015, employee health plan members' coinsurance payments depended on their choice of provider—10% co-pay if the provider was participating in BSWQA and was in network for the third-party administrator, 50% if the provider was in network for the third-party administrator but did not participate in BSWQA, and 70% if the provider was out of network for the third-party administrator. The incentive this structure provides to seek out providers who are both in network for the third-party administrator and participating in BSWQA is believed to be responsible for the increase seen in 2015 in the number of BSWH–North Texas employees with a BSWQA PCP.

Accountable Care Organizations: Legal Considerations*,†

ACOs received a degree of favorable legal and antitrust consideration by participating in MSSP and following other

* The author wishes to thank Matthew D. Jenkins, Hunton & Williams, LLP, for his assistance with the clinical integration checklist and James Pinna, Hunton & Williams, LLP, for his assistance with the summaries of the federal anti-kickback statute and Stark law. The author also wishes to recognize the significant role played by attorneys from Hunton & Williams, LLP and Norton Rose Fulbright in structuring BSWQA and providing ongoing advice to assist BSWQA to comply with applicable law.
† This section is intended to be a summary of legal issues created by the formation and operation of ACOs. It should not be construed as legal advice. Competent counsel should be consulted with respect to applicability of legal requirements in particular situations.

ACO-related provisions in the ACA. Yet the fact that they can
bring together otherwise competing health care providers,
who are referral sources for other members of the ACO,
or combinations of for-profit and tax-exempt not-for-profit
entities, means that careful attention needs to be paid during
their formation and operation to comply with antitrust laws,
statutes, and regulations related to participation in federal
health care programs; legal requirements for tax-exempt organizations; and state insurance laws. Further complicating the
issue is the fact that compliance with some of these laws may
create tension with being in compliance with others. It is
hardly surprising, therefore, that one of the frequently cited
hurdles to ACO formation is uncertainty about the legality of
their formation and operation [50]. This section summarizes
some of the laws most relevant to ACOs, providing real-world
examples of how they can impact an ACO's operation. It is
worth emphasizing early on, however, that the complexity of
the laws and their application to ACOs means that one of the
most important "lessons learned" that BSWQA has to share
is the value of involving competent legal counsel in both the
formation and ongoing operation of an ACO.

Antitrust

Antitrust laws seek to preserve competition, based on the
assumption that a competitive market controls cost and motivates high quality. Physicians and other professionals are subject to antitrust laws [91], so alignment of competing health care
providers into an ACO can trigger applicability of the antitrust
laws, especially if the ACO negotiates payment rates on behalf
of its independent participants. This does not, however, mean
that such arrangements necessarily violate the antitrust laws:
the Federal Trade Commission (FTC) and Department of Justice
(DOJ) have issued a number of joint statements addressing
arrangements in the health care industry [92] that recognize
that, under certain circumstances, combinations of otherwise

competing providers can create pro-competitive efficiencies by lowering costs and improving quality of care provided. These statements create "safety zones" that protect combinations of providers that meet certain conditions from antitrust scrutiny and challenge. Since lowering costs and improving quality of care were the motivations for the original conception of the ACO [12], these organizations may fit within these safety zones. Moreover, even an ACO that falls outside the established safety zones does not necessarily violate antitrust law; it is merely subject to greater scrutiny and so may be called on to demonstrate that it does, in fact, create pro-competitive efficiencies. The joint statements that are most applicable to ACOs are summarized in Table 3.2.

BSWQA is a multiprovider network, including physicians, hospitals, and other health care providers along the care continuum. As a result, it does not fit within the Joint Statement 8 safety zone for financially integrated physician-only networks. It also did not initially participate in MSSP, and so was not eligible for the safety zone established to encourage the formation and participation of ACOs in this program. As such, and like many physician-hospital ACOs, BSWQA falls into the less clear-cut area where the potential for antitrust violations is evaluated based on the balance between the anticompetitive effects of network formation and pro-competitive efficiencies (reduced costs and increased quality). Factors taken into account in this analysis include whether the network is financially or clinically integrated and whether it is exclusive or nonexclusive [92]. While BSWQA is not currently financially integrated and has not placed full financial risk on either physicians or hospitals, it can demonstrate essentially all the factors indicative of clinical integration summarized in Table 3.3. It is also nonexclusive, as BSWQA providers are not prohibited from participating in competing ACOs or negotiating individually with payers [95]. In fact, BSWQA's current contractual arrangements with payers require BSWQA participants to have a direct, individual agreement with the

Table 3.2 Summary of the FTC and DOJ Joint Statements of Enforcement Policy in Health Care Most Relevant to ACOs

Joint Statement 8: Physician Network Joint Ventures

Safety zone: Physician networks of a certain size that share substantial financial risk
 	
 Criteria:
 	
 1. Share substantial financial risk
    – *For example*:
      • Capitation
      • Provision of services for a predetermined percentage of a premium or revenue
      • Significant financial incentives for network physicians to achieve specified cost containment goals as a group
      • Bundled payments for a complex or extended course of treatment that requires substantial coordination between physicians in different specialties offering complementary services, and for which cost of the course of treatment for an individual patient can vary greatly due to factors beyond the physicians' control
 	
 2. Constitute ≤20% of the relevant market if the network is exclusive *or* ≤30% of the relevant market if the network is nonexclusive
    – *The relevant market consists of the physicians in each specialty with active hospital privileges who practice in the geographic market*
      • (Note that this statement provides little guidance on what constitutes a "geographic market.")
      • In the context of an ACO, the relevant market depends on the range of services offered by the ACO, and the definition of the "primary service area" from the ACO statement (below) may apply.
    – *Factors that indicate a network is nonexclusive*:
      • There are competing networks or managed care plans with adequate physician participation in the market.

Table 3.2 (*Continued*)   Summary of the FTC and DOJ Joint Statements of Enforcement Policy in Health Care Most Relevant to ACOs

- Physicians in the network participate in or contract with other networks and managed care plans (or there is evidence of their willingness and incentive to do so).

- Physicians in the network earn substantial revenue from other networks or through individual contracts with managed care plans.

- No indication of significant de-participation from other networks and managed care plans.

- No indication of coordination among physicians regarding price or other competitively significant terms of participation in other networks or managed care plans.

- No other provisions significantly restricting the ability or willingness of the physicians to join other networks or contract individually with managed care plans.

Clinically integrated physician networks

Networks that are clinically integrated are not treated as being in per se violation of the antitrust laws, but are analyzed in a manner that takes into account the pro-competitive efficiencies of the network and looks at whether the joint contracting efforts of the network and other collateral agreements are "subordinate to and reasonably necessary to achieve these objectives."

Criteria:

The FTC and DOJ have not issued a definitive list of criteria that need to be met to establish clinical integration.

1. Joint Statement 8 provides that clinical integration likely to produce pro-competitive efficiencies can be demonstrated by implementation of an active and ongoing program to evaluate and modify physician practice patterns and create a high degree of interdependence and cooperation among the physicians to control costs and ensure quality, which may include:

Continued

Table 3.2 (*Continued*)   Summary of the FTC and DOJ Joint Statements of Enforcement Policy in Health Care Most Relevant to ACOs

> – Establishing mechanisms to monitor and control utilization of health care services that are designed to control costs and assure quality of care
>
> – Selectively choosing network physicians who are likely to further the efficiency objectives
>
> – Significant investment of capital, monetary and human, in the necessary infrastructure and capability to achieve the claimed efficiencies
>
> 2. The FTC advisory opinion to MedSouth, Inc. [94] states that "the test of [clinical] integration is what the participants, through the network, actually do—i.e., how they use these tools to create cooperation and interdependence in their provision of medical care, thereby facilitating their efforts to jointly reduce unnecessary costs, improve quality of care, and otherwise increase their efficiency in the provision of medical care."
>
> 3. Other factors that have been considered by the FTC in advisory opinions determining whether providers were sufficiently clinically integrated to permissibly engage in collective fee negotiation with third-party payers are summarized in the clinical integration checklist developed by BSWQA and shown in Table 3.3.

Joint Statement 9: Multiprovider Networks

Safety zone: None

Joint Statement 9 applies to combinations of providers that are not limited to physicians. Because of the wide variety of networks that can potentially be formed, the FTC and DOJ have not defined a safety zone for multiprovider networks.

Analysis for antitrust violations

Similar to the safety zone and the clinical integration analyses above for physician networks, factors considered include:

■ Whether the network is either financially or clinically integrated

Table 3.2 (*Continued*) Summary of the FTC and DOJ Joint Statements of Enforcement Policy in Health Care Most Relevant to ACOs

■ Whether the network is exclusive or nonexclusive ■ The balance between the anticompetitive effects and pro-competitive efficiencies (reduced costs and increased quality) Joint Statement 9 also introduces the "messenger model," which avoids the need for horizontal agreements on price or price-related terms by using an agent to pass information between payers and individual members of the network, without sharing competitively sensitive information between members of the network. ■ Avoids collective bargaining on behalf of competing members within the network ■ Avoids creating or facilitating agreement among competing members within the network on prices or price-related terms
ACO Statement (issued by FTC and DOJ in connection with Medicare Shared Savings Program)

Safety zone: ACOs participating in MSSP that have ≤30% of the services in each primary service area
 	
Criteria:
 	
1. Have ≤30% of the services in each primary service area.
 	
  – The "primary service area" is defined as "the lowest number of postal zip codes from which the [ACO participant] draws at least 75 percent of its [patients]" [93]
 	
  – "Services" are defined as:
 	
  • For physicians: Primary specialty
 	
  • For inpatient facilities: Major diagnostic category for inpatient services
 	
  • For outpatient facilities: Outpatient categories of services defined by CMS

Continued

Table 3.2 (*Continued*) Summary of the FTC and DOJ Joint Statements of Enforcement Policy in Health Care Most Relevant to ACOs

2. Hospitals and ambulatory surgery centers must participate on a nonexclusive basis.

Analysis for ACO contracts outside of MSSP

Contracts with private payers outside MSSP are considered "reasonably necessary to an ACO's primary purpose of improving health care delivery"; thus, provided the ACO uses the same governance and leadership structure and clinical and administrative processes in the private payer context as in the MSSP, joint contracting will be evaluated through weighing the anticompetitive effects against the pro-competitive efficiencies.

Source: Department of Justice and Federal Trade Commission, Statements of antitrust enforcement policy in health care, 1996, http://www.justice.gov/atr/public/guidelines/0000.htm; Federal Trade Commission and Department of Justice, Statement of antitrust enforcement policy regarding accountable care organizations participating in the Medicare Shared Savings Program, 76 *Fed Reg* 67026–67031 (October 28, 2011).

particular payer. Furthermore, like other ACOs that fall outside the safety zones created by the FTC and DOJ, BSWQA shares many characteristics with the hypothetical, non–safety zone provider network described by the FTC and DOJ in the joint statements as one that they would consider to be "structured to achieve its [pro-competitive] efficiencies through a high degree of interdependence and cooperation among its physician participants [and that the] price agreement, under these circumstances, is subordinate to and reasonably necessary to achieve these objectives," and so would not challenge formation or operation [92]. These characteristics include:

- Formation with the purpose of working to reduce costs and maintain or improve the quality of care
- Implementation of systems to establish goals relating to quality and appropriate utilization by participants, to develop and implement practice standards and protocols

Table 3.3   BSWQA Checklist of Clinical Integration Standards (developed from FTC/DOJ Joint Statement 8 and FTC advisory opinions)

1. Implementation of systems to establish goals relating to quality and appropriate utilization of services by network's participants
2. Regular evaluation of both individual participants' and network's aggregate performance with respect to network's established goals
3. Modification of individual network participants' actual practices, where necessary, based on evaluations against established goals
4. Performance of:
a. Case management
b. Preauthorization
c. Concurrent review of inpatient stays
d. Retrospective review of inpatient stays
5. Adoption and implementation of clinical practice guidelines and performance goals relating to treatment, quality, and appropriate use of services provided by network participants
a. Significant number of practice standards and clinical protocols developed
b. Significant number of practice standards and clinical protocols deployed to network participants and governing treatment and utilization of services by network participants
c. Active review of the care rendered by each network participant in light of adopted practice standards and clinical protocols to determine compliance by individual network participants
6. Clinical information system to measure, monitor, send, and receive individual network participant performance and aggregate network performance, including, without limitation, compliance with clinical protocols
7. Established procedures to modify network participant behavior and assure adherence to network standards and protocols
8. Limitation of network participation through selective processes

Continued

Table 3.3 (*Continued*)   BSWQA Checklist of Clinical Integration Standards (developed from FTC/DOJ Joint Statement 8 and FTC advisory opinions)

9. Procedures contemplating remedial actions up to and including the possibility of expulsion from network for noncompliant network participants based on routine monitoring of compliance with clinical protocols and guidelines
10. Significant investments in network's infrastructure and operations in terms of monetary and human capital, including, without limitation, appreciable time spent in developing network's practice standards and protocols
11. Obligation of continued investment by network participants in time spent reviewing and updating network's standards and protocols
12. Requirement that network participants provide care to contracted covered lives with a high degree of interdependence and cooperation with other network participants
13. Necessity of joint contracting to achieve efficiencies
14. Requirement of in-network referrals
15. Absence of ability to exercise significant market power

governing treatment and utilization of services, and to regularly evaluate performance with respect to these standards and goals

■ Modification of individual participants' actual practices, where necessary, based on those evaluations, with the potential for remedial action or exclusion from the network for participants who do not comply with the standards and protocols

■ Case management

■ Investment of capital to purchase or develop information technology to gather, analyze, and report individual and aggregate data on the cost, quantity, and nature of services provided, as well as on quality of care and patient satisfaction measures

■ Employment of directors and support staff to perform the network's function and coordinate patient care

Physicians who are in an ACO know that to be successful in improving quality and reducing cost, retention of patients within the network is important. Practitioners cannot easily manage and direct the care of patients who are treated outside of the network. Retention of patients within the network is regarded as a sign of clinical integration by the FTC, yet efforts to retain the patients in network can raise concerns about self-referral provisions in the Stark law and anti-kickback statute discussed below.

Medicare Shared Savings Program

The MSSP [96] was established through the ACA [14], holding ACOs accountable for the quality and cost of services provided to Medicare patients and entitling the ACOs to share in any savings generated for the Medicare program. MSSP is intended to encourage organizations to form ACOs and invest in infrastructure and redesign of care processes to improve the quality and efficiency of care. The ACA specifies the types and arrangements of providers that can form an MSSP ACO and specifies certain capabilities and structural elements for participation [96]. Further criteria are specified under the regulations issued by CMS to implement MSSP [97], and as directed by the ACA, CMS has established performance measures and standards to assess the quality of care furnished by the ACOs, with regard to (1) clinical processes and outcomes, (2) patient and caregiver experience of care, and (3) utilization of services [96, 97].

BSWQA was first envisioned as participating in MSSP. This plan ran into a practical problem, however, in that MSSP requires patient attribution to be based on the physician's tax identification (TIN) number. Since some of the BSWQA physicians practice in groups that shared a single TIN for billing purposes and included physicians not participating in BSWQA, this would have put the ACO at risk for patients predominantly seeing a physician who was not participating in BSWQA's

clinical integration activities, risks, and rewards [72, 98].
BSWQA therefore directed its early focus toward private managed care contracts that offered opportunities for shared
savings. In 2015, BSWQA started participating in MSSP,
addressing the problem that TIN numbers continue to be used
for patient attribution through the practical measure of limiting
participation to primary care practices that include only
BSWQA physicians [72].

Participation in Federal Health Care Programs

Anti-Kickback Statute

The federal anti-kickback statute (AKS) prohibits the knowing
and willful offer, payment, solicitation, or receipt of any
remuneration, directly or indirectly, overtly or covertly, in cash
or in kind, to induce or reward referrals of items or services
reimbursable by a federal health care program [99]. The AKS
carries both criminal and civil penalties, including exclusion
from participation in federal health care programs, and is
violated even if the inducement of referrals of Medicare or
Medicaid patients is only *one purpose* of the arrangement,
among other, appropriate purposes [100, 101].

The AKS does, however, include statutory exceptions that
identify certain types of remuneration that are not prohibited;
additionally, safe harbor regulations identify certain transactions that are not subject to prosecution under the AKS [102].
Failing to meet all the criteria of a specific statutory exception
or safe harbor does not necessarily mean that a transaction
violates the AKS; however, such a transaction may be subject to closer scrutiny and may be found to violate the AKS
[103]. Advisory opinions issued by the Office of the Inspector
General (OIG) provide useful insight into how the OIG is
currently reviewing certain arrangements under the AKS and
are helpful to individuals and organizations engaging in transactions that need to be structured carefully to avoid running

afoul of the AKS. Making a good faith effort to comply with the safe harbor requirements and to incorporate positive features and avoid problematic features outlined by the OIG is important in the context of the AKS because the statute requires an individual or entity to "knowingly and willfully" violate its provisions.

The AKS is relevant to ACOs when they involve the transfer of value between referral sources. As such, these transactions within an ACO need to be structured to fit within a statutory exception or safe harbor to minimize the risk of an AKS challenge. Two important exceptions and safe harbors in the context of ACOs are those covering bona fide employment arrangements (which protect payments from the employer to the employee) and personal services and management con-tracts (which protect payments for such services made under a signed written agreement that meets the safe harbor require-ments) [104, 105]. These exceptions and safe harbors enable BSWQA to reimburse physicians, such as medical directors and committee chairs, for services rendered directly to the organization even when they are not directly employed by the organization. In such arrangements, signed contractual agreements meeting the safe harbor requirements have been executed between BSWQA and the independent physicians.

One of the hallmarks of arrangements that violate the AKS and the Stark law (discussed below) are arrangements where compensation fluctuates based on the volume or value of referrals. BSWQA's distributions of shared savings to its physician participants are carefully structured to avoid any consideration of volume or value of referrals. For example, the specialists in BSWQA divide the specialty share of shared savings equally regardless of the volume of patients seen or the charges of services to those patients.

In 2011, CMS and the OIG issued waivers of the AKS for ACOs participating in MSSP. These are discussed below, together with the waivers issued for other applicable laws.

Stark Law

The federal Stark law generally prohibits a physician from making a referral for "designated health services" (DHSs) (including, among other things, clinical laboratory services, radiology services, physical and occupational therapy services, and inpatient and outpatient hospital services) for a Medicare beneficiary if the physician has a financial relationship with the entity furnishing the DHS—unless that relationship meets one of the statutory or regulatory exceptions [106]. The Stark law also prohibits the provider of those services from billing Medicare for them. A financial relationship can take the form of a direct or indirect ownership interest or a compensation arrangement. Unlike the AKS safe harbors, a financial relationship that fails to satisfy *all* the requirements of a statutory or regulatory exception violates the Stark law if referrals of Medicare patients are made. Furthermore, there is no requirement that the violation be "knowing or willful." As such, ACOs like BSWQA that involve both physicians and providers of designated health services (e.g., hospitals) need to pay close attention to the Stark law and the criteria for its exceptions.

The Stark law exceptions most applicable in the ACO context are those addressing bona fide employment relationships, personal services relationships, and physician incentive plans [107, 108].

The exception for physician incentive plans, defined as "any compensation between a designated health services entity (or downstream contractor) and a physician or physician group that may directly or indirectly have the effect of reducing or limiting services furnished with respect to individuals enrolled with the entity" [109], permits the physician's compensation to be determined in a manner that takes into account the volume or value of any referrals or other business generated (through such mechanisms as withhold pools, capitation, and bonuses), provided the necessary conditions are met.

Civil Monetary Penalties Statute

The so-called civil monetary penalties statute (CMP law) prohibits a hospital or critical access hospital from knowingly making a direct or indirect payment to a physician as an inducement to reduce or limit services provided to Medicare or Medicaid patients who are under the direct care of the physician [110]. Penalties include a civil monetary penalty of $2,000 for each patient for whom payment is made in violation of the statute. The CMP law may apply to payments made within an ACO to the extent that these are considered direct or indirect payments by a hospital to a physician to reduce or limit services.

Over the years, hospitals have sought ways to reduce the cost and improve the quality of services provided to patients and have attempted to engage physicians in those efforts through a variety of means. One of these is "gainsharing," defined as sharing a portion of the savings achieved by the hospitals with the physicians who participated in efforts to reduce the cost of services. An early OIG special advisory opinion indicated that such gainsharing programs fall under jurisdiction of the CMP law [111], even if the cost savings are achieved through reductions in services that are not medically necessary, and a number of other advisory opinions have approved specific gainsharing arrangements. These advisory opinions can only be relied on by the requestor, but provide insight into how the OIG is viewing particular arrangements.

In a 2008 advisory opinion, the OIG identified both areas of concern that could raise issues under a gainsharing arrangement and features that could provide sufficient protection against fraud and abuse [112], summarized in Table 3.4.

In ACOs that involve physicians and hospitals, like BSWQA, structuring the arrangement to fit within the parameters of an OIG advisory opinion on gainsharing can help avoid a challenge under the CMP law—although the only certain way

Table 3.4   High-Risk and Protective Features of Gainsharing Plans

Features of a Gainsharing Plan That Raise Concerns	Features of a Gainsharing Plan That Protect against Fraud and Abuse
■ Stinting on patient care (withholding of medically necessary services)	■ Specific cost savings actions and the resulting savings are clearly and separately identified and sufficiently transparent to allow public scrutiny and individual physician accountability
■ "Cherry picking" healthy patients and steering sicker patients to hospitals that do not offer such arrangements	■ Implementation of the recommendations does not adversely affect patient care
■ Payments in exchange for patient referrals	■ The amounts paid under the arrangement are calculated based on all procedures performed, regardless of patient's insurance coverage, subject to the cap on payment for federal health care program procedures
	■ The procedures are not disproportionately performed on federal health care program beneficiaries
	■ The arrangement protects against improper service reductions by using objective historical and clinical measures to create baseline thresholds beyond which no savings accrue
	■ The hospital and the physician groups provide written disclosures of the arrangement to patients whose care may be affected

Table 3.4 (*Continued*) High-Risk and Protective Features of Gainsharing Plans

	■ Financial incentives are reasonably limited in duration and amount
	■ Profits are distributed on a per capita basis, mitigating any incentive for an individual physician to generate disproportionate cost savings

of avoiding such a challenge is receipt of a favorable OIG advisory opinion on the specific arrangement. While BSWQA has not sought an advisory opinion to this point, it regularly consults in-house and outside legal counsel on arrangements that have the potential for raising issues under the CMP law, as well as AKS and the Stark law.

The Medicare Access and CHIP Reauthorization Act of 2015 (MACRA) amends the CMP law to indicate that the prohibited payments from the hospital to the physician are those that are an inducement to reduce the provision of *medically necessary* services [113]. This change is effective for payments made after April 16, 2015. Since many gainsharing arrangements seek to eliminate medically unnecessary services, this change will likely significantly increase the prevalence of such arrangements.

ACO Waivers

The breadth of the AKS, Stark law, and CMP law raises concerns that they might stifle the formation and operation of ACOs. To encourage participation in MSSP, the OIG and CMS issued five waivers from applicability of these laws for certain arrangements involving ACOs participating in MSSP [114]. These waivers cover (1) ACO preparticipation, (2) ACO participation, (3) shared savings distribution, (4) compliance with the Stark law, and (5) patient incentives. Table 3.5 summarizes the main purposes and features of these waivers.

Table 3.5 Summary of the Five ACO Waivers

ACO Preparticipation Waiver

■ Covers arrangements that predate the ACO's participation in MSSP
 	
■ Offers a one-time waiver from applicability of the AKS, Stark law, and CMP law for 1 year prior to the ACO's targeted date for participating in MSSP, ending on the date:
 	
  1. The ACO enters into a participation agreement in the year targeted
 	
  2. The ACO's application is denied
 	
  3. The application is due if the ACO has not submitted an application, although in this case the ACO may seek an extension until the next application due date
 	
■ Requirements:
 	
  – Good faith intent to develop an ACO that will participate in MSSP
 	
  – Documented diligent steps to develop an ACO that would be eligible to participate in MSSP
 	
  – Documented decision by the ACO's governing body that the arrangement is reasonably related to the purposes of MSSP
 	
    • Promoting accountability for the quality, cost, and overall care for a Medicare population
 	
    • Managing and coordinating care for Medicare beneficiaries through an ACO
 	
    • Encouraging investment in infrastructure and redesigned care processes for high-quality and efficient service delivery for patients, including Medicare beneficiaries
 	
  – Public disclosure of the arrangement
 	
  – Submission of an application to participate in MSSP *or* of a statement describing why it was unable to submit an application, before the last available application due date in the targeted year

Table 3.5 (*Continued*)   Summary of the Five ACO Waivers

ACO Participation Waiver
■ Covers arrangements involving the ACO, one or more of the ACO's participants or providers and suppliers, or a combination thereof, from the date the ACO becomes an MSSP participant to 6 months following the earlier of: 1. The expiration of the MSSP participation agreement 2. The date on which the ACO voluntarily terminates the MSSP participation agreement ■ Requirements: – The ACO remains in good standing with MSSP – The ACO meets the MSSP requirements for governance, leadership, and management – A duly authorized and bona fide determination by the ACO's governing body that the arrangement is reasonably related to the purposes of MSSP (defined as above) – A documented and publicly disclosed description of the arrangement and the date and manner of the governing body's authorization of the arrangement ■ May provide some protection for incentives or other arrangements targeting the ACO's commercial patients, as CMS and OIG recognize that such arrangements have the potential to be "reasonably related to the purposes of the Shared Savings Program" [114, 115]

Shared Savings Distribution Waiver
■ Covers distributions or uses of shared savings earned by the ACO ■ Requirements: – The ACO becomes and remains a participant in good standing in MSSP – The shared savings are earned through MSSP during the term of its MSSP participation agreement, even if distribution occurs after the end of the MSSP participation agreement

Continued

Table 3.5 (*Continued*) Summary of the Five ACO Waivers

– The shared savings are
 	
  1. Distributed among the ACO's participants and its providers and suppliers or individuals or entities that were ACO participants or providers and suppliers in the year in which the shared savings were earned
 	
  2. Used for activities that are reasonably related to MSSP
 	
– For purposes of the CMP law, distributions by a hospital directly or indirectly to a physician are not made knowingly to induce the physician to reduce or limit medically necessary items or services to patients under the physician's direct care

Compliance with Stark Law Waiver

■ Applies to any financial relationship between or among the ACO and the ACO's participants or providers and suppliers that implicates the Stark law
 	
■ Waives scrutiny under the AKS and CMP law for ACO arrangements that use existing Stark law exceptions
 	
■ Applies from the date the ACO becomes an MSSP participant to 6 months following the earlier of:
 	
  1. The expiration of the MSSP participation agreement
 	
  2. The date on which the ACO voluntarily terminates the MSSP participation agreement
 	
■ Requirements:
 	
  – The ACO becomes and remains a participant in good standing in MSSP
 	
  – The financial relationship is reasonably related to the purposes of MSSP (defined as above)
 	
  – The financial relationship fully complies with an exception to the Stark law

Table 3.5 (*Continued*)   Summary of the Five ACO Waivers

Patient Incentives Waiver

■ Applies to the AKS and the section of the CMP law that prohibits offering or transferring remuneration to a Medicare or Medicaid beneficiary that the person knows or should know is likely to influence such person to order or receive from a particular provider, practitioner, or supplier any item or service for which payment may be made under Medicare or Medicaid

■ Recognizes that ACOs need to engage patients in better managing their own health care, including obtaining preventive care and complying with treatment plans for chronic conditions

■ Covers items or services provided by an ACO or its ACO participants or providers and suppliers to Medicare or Medicaid beneficiaries for free or below fair market value, starting from the date the ACO enters into an MSSP participation agreement and ending 6 months after the earlier of:

1. The expiration of the MSSP participation agreement

2. The date on which the ACO voluntarily terminates the MSSP participation agreement provided that the beneficiary may keep items received or receive the remainder of services initiated before termination from MSSP

■ Requirements:

– The ACO becomes and remains a participant in good standing in MSSP

– There is a reasonable connection between the item or service and the medical care of the beneficiary

– The items or services

1. Are preventive care items or services

2. Advance one or more of the following goals: (a) adherence to a treatment regime, (b) adherence to a drug regime, (c) adherence to a follow-up care plan, or (d) management of a chronic disease

Source: Department of Health and Human Services, Centers for Medicare and Medicaid Services, and Office of the Inspector General, Medicare Program, Final waivers in connection with the Shared Savings Program, 76 *Fed Reg* 67991–68010 (November 2, 2011).

Tax Exemption

ACOs may include entities that are exempt from federal income tax under Section 501(c)(3) of the Internal Revenue Code. BSWQA is treated as a taxable entity even though it is wholly owned by hospitals that are tax exempt. Tax-exempt entities must be operated exclusively for one or more exempt purposes—in the case of health care providers, the charitable purpose is the promotion of health. An organization is not operated exclusively for exempt purposes if its net earnings inure in whole or in part to the benefit of private shareholders or individuals ("private inurement") [116]. It must also serve a public rather than a private interest and may not be organized or operated for the benefit of private interests such as designated individuals, the creator of the organization or his family, shareholders of the organization, or persons controlled, directly or indirectly, by such private interests ("impermissible private benefit") [117].

Tax-exempt members of an ACO may provide start-up or ongoing financial assistance to the ACO or engage in financial transactions with one or more nonexempt members of the ACO, both of which have the potential to raise private inurement or impermissible private benefit issues.

Because uncertainty regarding the impact participating in an ACO might have on a health care provider's tax-exempt status could raise a barrier to organizations' willingness to form ACOs or participate in MSSP, the Internal Revenue Service (IRS) issued Notice 2011-20 [118], providing guidance on this issue. While the IRS indicated that the determination of whether an exempt organization's participation in MSSP resulted in private inurement or impermissible private benefit would be made on a case-by-case basis, it identified a number of conditions under which it would not expect to find such problems. These include the exempt organization having a written agreement, negotiated at arm's length, with the ACO; current participation of the ACO in MSSP; proportionality of the exempt organization's economic benefits derived from the ACO to the benefits or contributions it provides; proportionality and equality in value of any ownership interest the exempt organization has in the ACO to its capital contributions; proportionality of ACO returns of capital, allocations, and distributions to ownership interest; and fair market value of all contracts and transactions between the exempt organization and the ACO, and between the ACO and its participants and other parties [118]. BSWQA has made considerable efforts to comply with these conditions through consulting with legal counsel and third-party valuation consultants.

Furthermore, in the absence of private inurement and impermissible private benefit, MSSP payments received by the exempt organization from the ACO are considered derived from activities that lessen the burdens of government (i.e., charitable activities) and therefore are not subject to unrelated business income tax [118]. However, when ACOs engage in activities unrelated to MSSP, such as negotiating with private insurance companies on behalf of unrelated parties, which are not considered charitable, these activities may be inconsistent with the organization's tax exemption or be subject to unrelated business income tax [118].

State Insurance Law

The types of payment that an ACO receives from payers or employers, or the taking of "downside risk" in payment arrangements with payers and employers, may trigger issues under state insurance law. For example, under some state laws, capitation arrangements in which an ACO receives a per patient per month payment to provide the full range of services to enrollees could be construed as the ACO engaging in the business of insurance, requiring a license and the establishment of financial reserves. In addition, many states have "any willing provider" laws, which require a managed care organization to include in its network all providers meeting certain criteria. These laws, if applicable to ACOs, could conflict with the intent of ACOs, like BSWQA, to only recruit physicians committed to be *accountable* to the mission of improving quality, reducing cost, and clinically integrating. Insurance laws and regulations and guidance from state insurance departments vary from state to state, so ACOs should consider the applicability of state insurance laws to their various payment and network formation arrangements.

In conclusion, the formation and operation of an ACO raises issues under myriad complex laws and regulations, with specific provisions that may be contradictory. For example, one of the factors that can help demonstrate clinical integration for antitrust law purposes requires ACO participants to keep referrals within the ACO network—something that can create issues under the AKS and Stark law. For ACOs participating in MSSP, the relevant enforcement agencies have issued statements, waivers, and guidance that help resolve these issues—including the ACO statement for antitrust law; the ACO waivers for the AKS, Stark law, and CMP law; and the IRS's Notice 2011-20 regarding tax-exempt entities participating in MSSP. Yet careful attention still needs to be paid not only to the specific requirements of these various safety zones, waivers, and exceptions, but also to any ACO activities that are unrelated to MSSP.

Governance and Organization

Physician Leadership in Accountable Care Organizations

Success in ACOs' mission to improve population health and reduce costs of care will require fundamental changes to the way health care is delivered. Physicians are at the center of health care delivery, making their buy-in to the *accountable* process essential. While it is too early to judge the success of the various ACO models, evidence from multispecialty medical groups with shared leadership structures (in which multiple stakeholders, including hospitals, medical groups, and insurers, act as partners, sharing both leadership and rewards or penalties earned) is impressive. Groups such as the Mayo Clinic, Kaiser Permanente, Intermountain Healthcare, and Geisinger Health System—that have achieved superior outcomes [119]— demonstrate the importance of integrating physician and administrative leadership. Furthermore, since most care begins with a physician order, physicians are responsible for at least 75% of the cost incurred within health care organizations, making them key players in any initiatives like ACOs that target both quality and efficiency of care [120]. Physicians are well suited to addressing these "value" problems—the need to increase quality while decreasing costs [121]—because they can influence both elements [122].

Physician leaders can provide the clinical knowledge about health care quality and safety that nonclinician executives may lack [123] and can help bridge the communication gap between hospital leaders and frontline clinicians [124]. Specifically with respect to the latter, physician leaders' clinical experience can help them recognize and meet some of the unique leadership challenges that health care organizations such as ACOs face. These include complexity due to patients requiring care within multiple "siloed" clinical areas, physician training and culture that makes them resist the collaboration and "followership" that are necessary parts of teamwork, and the urgency of the need to improve access, affordability, and quality of health care [125, 126]. Physician leadership can also reduce the perception that the motivation behind changes the organization calls for is strictly financial, rather than primarily patient care concerns—in turn reducing physician resistance and bolstering professionalism [124]. At the end of the day, the success of ACOs will depend greatly on the institution of fundamental *accountable* changes in physicians' daily practice to accomplish the transition from a fee-for-service to a value-based model.

Such changes will require not only organizational physician leadership in ACOs, but also physician peer leadership.

Within BSWQA, 18 of the 21 members of the board of managers, including the chair, are physicians, representing both employed and independent physician groups. The president, chief medical and medical information officers, and medical directors, as well as the majority of members and the chairs of all the governance committees (described below), are physicians, providing broad physician leadership for all aspects of BSWQA's operations.

Baylor Scott & White Quality Alliance Governance and Organization

BSWQA is a limited liability corporation wholly owned by BSWH. Its board of managers is physician led and includes 18 practicing physicians, two BSWH executives, and a community representative (who is also a Medicare beneficiary). The physician board members were initially selected by asking the member hospitals and affiliated medical practice groups to nominate physicians from their medical staffs who viewed the ACO approach positively, had reputations for delivering and advocating for high-quality, evidence-based care, and were well respected by their peers. The founding board of BSWQA approved its mission statement, "to achieve the highest quality and most cost-effective care possible for the patients that we serve through clinical integration" (Figure 3.3). The early focus was on recruiting physicians into the BSWQA network, and therefore needed several respected physician leaders able to spread the message about how the ACO could help improve quality and efficiency. AS BSWQA has matured, the board has evolved toward membership that provides special expertise in population management and is fully committed to the vision of the ACO. It can be expected that, over time, the skill sets needed, and therefore specific composition of the board, are likely to keep changing. What remains constant, however, is

Mission Statement
"Why we exist as an organization"

Baylor Scott & White Quality
Alliance's mission is to achieve the
highest quality and most cost
effective care possible for the patients
that we serve through clinical
integration

Figure 3.3 BSWQA Mission Statement.

the determination that BSWQA should remain physician led
and mission driven.

BSWQA executive leaders were drawn extensively from
within BSWH, ensuring that the new leadership had in-depth
knowledge of the system's operations, strengths, and weaknesses. The president of BSWQA, for example, in addition to
having 40 years of experience as a practicing family physician,
is a past vice president of health care improvement for BHCS
and spent 14 years as founding chairman of the board of
HTPN [72, 127]. The BSWQA chief medical and chief administrative officers similarly have many years of leadership experience within BSWH and, in fact, hold joint appointments—the
former as chief quality officer for HTPN and vice president for
chronic disease within BSWH and the latter as chief administrative officer for HTPN [72, 127]. This system-savvy leadership has been critical to integrating the priorities related to
population health and BSWQA's shared savings model with
other initiatives and transformations in which BSWH and its
employed physician groups are engaged. Without such integration, there is high risk of both needless duplication of effort
and delays related to competing priorities. By integrating
efforts, BSWQA and BSWH are reinforcing their collaborative
culture [72]. But while the ~1,800 employed physicians are
foundational in the BSWQA strategy, the organization also

seeks to integrate the many willing, independent physicians in the areas it serves into the accountable quality alliance.

Essential Baylor Scott & White Quality Alliance Committees

An extensive physician-led committee structure is responsible for creating policies, establishing and evaluating membership criteria, monitoring regulatory compliance and financial performance, and creating disease management and population management care delivery protocols and pathways within BSWQA. Table 3.6 outlines the primary functions of each major committee that reports directly to the board of managers.

Table 3.6 Functions of the BSWQA Committees

Committee	Function
Membership and standards	Create standards of membership and manage performance of all participants; NCQA-accepted credentialing of physicians and other providers, and standards for alliance with post–acute care providers and facilities.
Best care/clinical integration	Multidisciplinary creation and monitoring of quality and efficiency of care paths across continuum of care; chronic disease management; transitional care management. This committee has almost 25 specialty subcommittees, each responsible for specialty-specific processes.
Compliance	Organizational adherence to regulatory requirements; assurance of rights and ethical care for patients served.
Finance, contracting, and compensation	Monitor financial performance of organization; create and adjudicate reward distribution; approve managed care contracts.
Population health information technology	Ensure electronic connectivity to support clinical integration and measure both quality and cost performance.

The Best Care/Clinical Integration (BC/CI) Committee is responsible for promoting evidence-based medicine and is comprised of practicing physicians, nurse administrators, and care coordination staff, all of whom are involved in the development and approval processes for clinical initiatives. The BC/CI Committee is multidisciplinary and subsequently segmented into 29 medical subcommittees, task forces, and councils, each of which is chaired by a physician leader. The chairperson populates the membership of his or her group to include representatives from BSWH as well as independent physicians. The groups listed in Table 3.7 report to the BC/CI Committee.

Role of Evidence-Based Medicine

Evidence-based medicine is "the integration of best research evidence with clinical expertise and patient values" [128]. Another way of phrasing this concept is that it requires delivery of the right care to the right patient at the right time. It includes avoiding underuse of necessary, effective treatments, avoiding overuse of unnecessary care, avoiding error, and making use of preference-sensitive care in accordance with individual patients' goals for treatment [129, 130]. It lies at the heart of any value-based payment mechanism—including an ACO's shared savings—that incorporates process-of-care measures among the quality metrics through which it assesses value. Measurement and feedback of performance of evidence-based care (either indirectly in the form of evidence-based process measures such as performance of annual HbA1c tests in patients with diabetes or directly in the form of outcome measures such as preventable readmissions to the hospital) are also important for driving continuous quality improvement. BSWQA leaders understand that one cannot manage or improve things that are not measured.

Barriers to the consistent practice of evidence-based medicine are manifold [131]. First, high-quality evidence is lacking in many areas of care—or if relevant studies have been

Table 3.7   Best Care Committee Subcommittees

Subcommittee members define evidence-based clinical protocols, establish the corresponding measures to evaluate performance, communicate and implement protocols and measures, and oversee performance improvement for BSWQA physicians within that specialty. These committees in turn report to the Best Care/CI Committee.	
■ Anesthesiology Subcommittee	■ Oncology Subcommittee
■ Asthma/COPD Council	■ Pain Management Task Force
■ Cardiovascular Subcommittee	■ Pathology Subcommittee
■ Colorectal Surgery Subcommittee	■ Pediatrics Subcommittee
■ Diabetes Council	■ Pharmacy and Therapeutics Subcommittee
■ Emergency Medicine Subcommittee	■ Post–Acute Care Council
■ Endocrinology Subcommittee	■ Primary Care Subcommittee
■ Gastroenterology Subcommittee	■ Pulmonary/Critical Care Subcommittee
■ General Surgery Subcommittee	■ Radiology Subcommittee
■ Heart Failure Task Force	■ Readmissions Reduction Council
■ Hospitalists Council	■ Rheumatology Subcommittee
■ Low Back Pain Task Force	■ Urology Subcommittee
■ Musculoskeletal Subcommittee	■ Vascular Subcommittee
■ Nephrology Subcommittee	■ Women's Health Subcommittee
■ Neurology Subcommittee	

conducted, often they have not been conducted in patients similar to the one for whom the physician is caring [131]. The lack of high-quality evidence is particularly great for patients of advanced age, patients with multiple or serious comorbidities, or patients of a racial or ethnic minority, who are frequently excluded from or underrepresented in the randomized controlled trials in which the efficacy of new treatments are tested [132, 133]. While large, rigorously conducted, population-based studies can provide valuable evidence of effectiveness in broader, real-world patient populations (and, if they are large enough, in specific subgroups who may have been excluded from randomized controlled trials), the large registries with detailed clinical data and long-term follow-up needed to provide this evidence are rare.

Second, comparative effectiveness evidence is lacking where multiple strategies to treat or manage the same condition are available [39]. This includes different treatment paths that offer similar survival but carry risks of different adverse events (or different timing of adverse events) that may be relevant to a patient's quality of life, as well as head-to-head comparisons of competing pharmaceuticals or devices.

Third, but most important, it is difficult to translate what evidence is available into actual practice. A commonly quoted estimate is that it takes an average of 17 years for research evidence to be integrated into clinical practice—although this average obscures the substantial complexity in measuring time lags, ignores variation in the underlying causes of the time lag, and assumes all time lags are bad (when, in fact, some might be related to establishing safety) [134]. One factor contributing to at least some time lags is that, for many of the clinical questions that have been studied, there is no single definitive study that clearly establishes the path supported by the evidence. Rather, there are multiple published reports, of variable quality and applicability to the physician's particular patient population, often with conflicting results. Few physicians have either the training in research methods or the time available to wade through the accumulated evidence, evaluate the quality of each study's methods—and thus the credibility of its results—and aggregate the results accordingly [131, 135]. Professional associations and organizations like the Cochrane Collaboration [136] attempt to alleviate this problem by convening panels of experts to review the evidence and compile it into clinical guidelines, or by having researchers conduct systematic reviews or meta-analyses to determine in what direction the weight of the evidence points. This has resulted in large numbers of evidence-based clinical guidelines and checklists. But there is substantial evidence that merely publishing guidelines or a meta-analysis has little impact on clinical practice [137], and even clear-cut initiatives such as the use of aspirin for patients suffering an acute myocardial infarction [138], hand hygiene [139], and the adult preventive services recommended by the U.S. Preventive Services Task Force [140] have taken far too long to be adopted into the daily routines of clinical care.

In BSWQA, this is where the Best Care Committee and its subcommittees come into play. This committee takes the available evidence—guidelines and published data, as well as existing data regarding patient care and outcomes—and distills it into care paths and protocols that can be implemented across the BSWQA care continuum. The Best Care Committee only passes protocols and care paths that are considered well evidenced. Additionally, it and its specialty subcommittees may adopt national initiatives that are well grounded in evidence, such as the Choosing Wisely® campaign [141]. The committee also only focuses on protocols that can be measured.

Mechanisms for implementation include order sets, alteration of the EHR to provide clinical decision support and collect structured data to enable reporting on related quality measures, and physician champions who can provide one-on-one education about why the particular change in practice is needed. The ACO also provides tools to help facilitate adoption of changes and the individual physicians' performance (and comparative performance to other BSWQA physicians) in achieving each measure. Yet guidelines and protocols alone cannot assure that evidence-based care will be *accountably* and reliably delivered.

How Data Drive Performance

Entities within BSWH have a long history of using performance measures to drive improvement [70, 71], and BSWQA was able to draw on this experience as it established its data analytics and reporting resources. The BSWQA Data Operations Group integrates data from the employed physician EHRs, the BSWH hospitals, and a full download of claims for contracted patients. Performance data are obtained from the resulting database. Essential steps in the successful use of data to drive performance are:

1. Identifying measures that are credible, relevant, and for which either data are available from an existing source or data collection is practicable. Within BSWQA, these measures originate from either primary care committees or specialty subcommittees and are approved by the Best Care Committee. Approved measures are introduced via newsletters, emails, website announcements, and video presentations. BSWQA members can access the complete protocol and measure list on the organization's secure member website.
2. Collecting, analyzing, and presenting the data.
   a. Depending on the type of measure chosen, substantial work may be required behind the scenes to ensure the correct data are included in the performance measurement: for process-of-care measures (such as annual HbA1c testing for patients with diabetes) this often requires careful determination of which patients fall within the eligibility criteria. For outcome measures (such as 30-day readmissions for patients hospitalized

with pneumonia), detailed data may have to be assembled from multiple different sources to properly capture not only the applicable patients and the outcome of interest, but also other relevant patient clinical and demographic data that are needed for risk adjustment to account for differences between providers and the case mix [142].

b. Once the data have been compiled and the analytic models developed and tested, a reporting format that is easily and intuitively interpreted by viewers, yet provides the necessary detail to be used to guide performance improvement, is needed. The BSWQA Best Care Committee has authorized three levels of performance reporting.

   i. *Organizational performance on a single initiative*
This report guides the Best Care Committee, the board, and the management team in defining key improvement opportunities related to quality and cost, and reflects overall organizational success.

   ii. *Regional comparative reports*
BSWQA is divided geographically into PODs and the comparative performance on initiatives uncovers opportunities for organizational support and improvement. Medical directors and BSWQA network field advisors attend regular POD meetings, where the transparent performance reports are discussed with specialists and referring PCPs reviewing each other's performance data.

   iii. *Individual physician performance reports*
These reports, called "data to the bedside" within BSWQA, are posted monthly on each physician's individual webpage and are discussed during "lunch-and-learn" sessions at the practice level led by regional physician champions. These reports form the basis for the BSWQA shared savings distributions.

3. Once the reports are distributed, the next step, especially the first few times physicians receive performance data, is convincing those who showed lower performance scores than they would have predicted for themselves that the data are valid and correct.

   a. It is essential that the data presented to the physicians be high-quality data and that appropriate adjustments for case mix are made. Frequent reactions to a low performance score are "The data must be wrong" and "Well, my patients are sicker than the other physicians' patients," as well as concern that the data might be used punitively. The quality of both the data and the analysis therefore needs to be as valid as possible, and errors must be corrected when they are identified because such errors compromise the credibility of not only the report on that measure, but also all the performance data being reported. Data are used for improvement purposes only, but unwillingness to improve in the face of persistent poor performance must carry consequences related to continued participation in the *accountable* network.

   b. BSWQA uses physician champions who meet one-on-one with member physicians to help them accept, first, the credibility of the reported data; second, the evidence supporting the practice on which performance is being measured (and its applicability to the physician's own patient population); and third, that the performance reports can help them find ways to provide better care for their patients.

An example of data-driven improvement within BSWQA comes from its Medicare Advantage (MA) contracts. The contracts offer BSWQA the opportunity to share in savings achieved when the total costs of care are lower than an agreed-on target. Both the target and the associated revenue CMS pays to the MA carrier are calculated according to the severity of illness in the contract population—defined as the risk adjustment factor (RAF) score. The accuracy of the RAF score depends on International Classification of Diseases (ICD-9) coding (performed by clinicians) of all conditions for all patients. The BSWQA RAF scores for their MA contract populations were initially low (implying to CMS that the population is relatively healthy, and the resultant CMS payment to the MA carrier was relatively low). While multiple reasons underlie the low BSWQA RAF scores, one was that physicians had not previously found value in coding "everything" wrong with each patient. By using certified coders to review claims before submission and instituting a physician education program that included the review of their individual RAF scores as well as identification of patients that likely had missed coding opportunities, the scores are now approaching the expected levels for the population served.

Care Coordination

One of the greatest challenges to improving the quality of and reducing the costs of care in the United States is the fragmented nature of the health care system. The fragmentation creates redundant diagnostic tests and procedures and conflicting treatments, as a patient moves from one siloed provider to another to obtain the care he or she needs. It also creates gaps and omissions at care transitions through which patients frequently fall, undoing much of the benefit of whatever care they had just received. An important function of an ACO is to reduce this fragmentation and create a well-integrated care experience. While some of this work lies on the technical side—for example, establishing HIE interoperability between the EHRs to facilitate timely sharing of patient information across the care continuum—a key component lies in care coordination.

BSWQA has invested heavily in care coordination resources (nurse care managers, medical assistant health coordinators, and social workers) and integrated these with existing resources within the hospitals and employed physician groups. These integrated resources cover all patients within the BSWQA contract population. In the SWH clinics practices, which are typically fairly large practices either affiliated with a hospital or set up as an outpatient department of a hospital, BSWQA care coordinators have been added to existing staff, but focus only on BSWQA patients within that practice. For a more detailed description of care coordination within BSWQA, see Chapter 5.

Will Accountable Care Organizations Work?

Will ACOs work? The jury is still out on this question. Although several ACOs, including BSWQA, have performed well to date, positive initial trends do not guarantee good long-term results. The only way to determine if ACOs work is to collect long-term data by which the effects of the various ACO models that have been implemented across the United States can be assessed. Preliminary results from MSSP ACOs show that 54% of these ACOs were able to reduce their spending relative to their benchmark in their first year, with 26% reducing spending sufficiently to qualify for shared savings (although 10% of these failed to satisfy the quality reporting requirements and so did not receive shared savings) [143]. Results from the Pioneer ACO model, which was designed for health systems with more experience assuming financial risk for patient populations, have also been mixed, showing some success in generating savings and improving performance on quality measures, but struggling to retain participants [144]. While the program yielded total savings of $96 million in its second year, paid $68 million to ACOs in shared savings, and showed a mean quality score improvement of 19%, as well as improved performance on 28 of 33 measures between performance years 1 and 2, only 40% to 55% of the participating ACOs earned shared savings in the first two years, and more than one-third of the ACOs had left the program by the end of year 2 [144]. What performance and patient outcomes might look like in the long term, however, remains very much in the balance. But while data may be lacking, opinions regarding the likely success or failure of ACOs abound.

Skeptics who doubt that ACOs will achieve the needed reductions in health care costs and spending, as well as the improved quality of care and population health, to bring the United States into line with other developed nations on health outcomes and costs [41], point to the similarities between ACOs and the integrated delivery networks (IDNs) introduced during the 1990s. IDNs failed as heavy financial losses were incurred by hospitals through purchases of physician practices, along with the networks' inability to align incentives across providers, piecemeal entry into capitated contracts with a few private insurers, and lack of infrastructure to manage risk [145]. Punitive "mother may I" utilization management systems and the use of gatekeepers also motivated resistance to managed care in the 1990s. Certainly, ACOs and managed care in that era have some similarities. Shared characteristics include their stated purpose of improving quality of care and population health while reducing costs, their focus on creating a care continuum, the use of centralized contracting for multiple providers in the network, the encouragement of horizontal and vertical consolidation of providers, and the emphasis on primary care in achieving the needed quality improvement and cost reduction [145]. The encouragement of consolidation runs the risk of creating large ACOs that dominate their markets by commanding high payments from insurers and marginalizing smaller providers—obviating the need for them to improve quality or reduce cost—which antitrust enforcement may be insufficient to prevent [146]. And, similar to the IDN's piecemeal entry into capitated contracts, providers within ACOs are typically also providing services for a large number or even a majority of their patients outside the ACO contracts, meaning they are dealing with diametrically opposed payment incentives: one that rewards cost containment and improved performance on chosen quality measures, and the other that rewards increased volume of services [146]. Without a dramatic increase in the number of ACO contracts from health insurance plans employing value-based payment mechanisms to tip the balance in favor of the quality improvement and cost containment incentives, this situation could prevent ACOs from succeeding. This is particularly true where their participating providers have "the incumbent's dilemma," wherein they have been very successful in fee-for-service settings and have little incentive to change [146]. Given that only 7% of physicians in a recent survey were enthusiastic about moving away from a fee-for-service reimbursement structure, this may prove to be a substantial barrier [66]. Recognizing this, the Department of Health and Human Services has announced plans to promote alternative payment models (see Chapter 3, Disruptive Effect of Volume to Value). In the interim, however, successful ACOs must demonstrate ambidexstrous skill required to thrive in both payment worlds.

The ACO model's emphasis on primary care to drive the needed changes is also problematic in that the supply of PCPs in the United States is both insufficient and unevenly geographically distributed for the population [145]. Furthermore, these physicians are unlikely to have the time available to provide the kind of care coordination envisioned within the ACO model for complex patients with multiple chronic conditions, unless a means of freeing up time they currently spend on low-risk patients and wellness visits can be implemented [145]. Other challenges of the ACO model that have been identified include the patient's freedom to seek care from any provider, which makes patient engagement and influence of quality and costs of care challenging; the lack of a standardized set of performance measures used across ACO contracts; reliance on retrospective annual shared savings payments that make securing capital to invest in care redesign and improvement difficult; and what may be unrealistic assumptions about the extent to which both physicians and patients will be *accountable* to change their behavior under the new model of care [147, 148]. Finally, the length of time ACOs may require to make meaningful impacts on costs and population health might be longer than either policy makers or providers are prepared to wait [146]; moreover, all savings represent lost income for someone, and affected stakeholders have in the past successfully blocked, weakened, or circumvented past efforts at cost control [38].

Advocates of ACOs point out that studies of similar provider-led delivery systems demonstrate that this model can achieve higher quality at reduced cost than the more typically fragmented care in most markets [149, 150]. They also argue that health care stakeholders will find ways to make ACOs succeed because the alternatives are not favorable for anyone. Most health care leaders know that the current system of care and financing must change. Unlike the failed efforts around IDNs and payment reforms in the 1990s, returning to the status quo is not an option: the inexorably rising health costs will force both public and private payers into cuts in provider payment rates, and with little data regarding performance on quality and cost measures available, these cuts are likely to be indiscriminate with respect to provider quality. Such cuts would potentially decrease both access to and quality of care available as providers either suffer financially, cease practice, or focus on increasing the volume of services they provide to make up for the decreases in payment [151]. Other differences from previous attempts at health care delivery reform include the HIT and data analytic capabilities now available, which facilitate data sharing and performance measurement and reporting in ways that were not previously possible, as well as the fact that, this time, the impetus behind the change came from CMS, which may be able to serve as a patron and protector of the restructuring [145].

While many factors will have to coincide for ACOs to achieve their stated aim of improving quality while reducing costs, the voluntary *accountability* of physicians, hospitals, and others who are willing to change patterns of care, follow evidence-based guidelines, avoid waste (which is revenue generating under fee-for-service reimbursement models), and improve based on performance data is critical. Changing from the fee-for-service to value-based payments is expected to help drive change, as behavioral economic realities such as financial incentives will take effect [152].

Until the long-term survival and performance of ACOs can be determined, however, health care stakeholders are faced with a choice between two sets of risks. They can commit to early adoption of the ACO concept, risking the necessary investment of population health resources in establishing the ACO infrastructure and the volume losses in accepting risk-based ACO contracts in a model of care that has not yet demonstrated value. In return for these risks, they have the opportunity to establish themselves in a dominant position within the market so that, if the ACO model succeeds, they are positioned to be skilled value providers for population health. From a clinical and administrative standpoint, this will require the ambidexterity described earlier in this chapter, in order to juggle both fee-for-service and value-based contracts.

Alternatively, they can wait for the data showing how successful ACOs are or are not succeeding. While this strategy avoids the risks inherent in investing in an unproven model of health care reform, it carries its own risk: if ACOs succeed, health care stakeholders who took the "wait and see" approach may well find themselves ill-equipped to compete with the early adopters and without a seat at the decision-making table. The choice must be made according to the organization's (or individual's) ability to absorb the potential short-term losses as well as the priority it places on the potential long-term gains. BSWQA, its physicians, and its hospitals have decided to seriously develop *accountability* for transforming care for the populations served.

Chapter 4

Patient Experience of Care

Main Points for Chapter

This chapter includes a discussion of:

- How consumerism drives accountability in health care
- The importance of data and pricing transparency in accountable care
- How technology, wellness, and patient self-management promote greater accountability in health care
- The use of quality metrics to allocate shared savings and facilitate better integration between hospital and ambulatory care

Responding to Consumerism through Accountable Care Organizations

Consumerism is a term that incorporates individuals' choices, economic incentives, purchasing decisions, and pursuit of their own well-being. Consumers historically have created or responded to major shifts in communication (cell phones), entertainment (web), transportation (electric cars), and banking (ATMs), just to name a few areas. Consumerism in health care is emerging as a powerful force demanding a patient-centric, patient-driven approach to health care, one that emphasizes better access to care, patient choice (e.g., of health plans, care providers, services, and treatments), and patient participation in decisions regarding care delivery and cost [153]. Health care consumerism will necessitate transparent availability of information so consumers who are not yet patients, and those who are under care currently, can be more informed about and more involved in medical decision-making processes [154]. ACOs, with their commitment to achieving the Triple Aim [1], particularly the aim of improving the patient experience of care, are uniquely positioned to foster greater patient involvement in their care through enhanced transparency of quality and cost data, communication by providers, better access, and a strong sense of *accountability* by providers to honor consumers' wishes, and bring them value, while delivering high-quality care.

Activated Consumers

Alice was very pleased as she walked out of her PCP's office. She had come for a second opinion after another physician suggested that her back pain, which had begun two days before when she was lifting groceries from her car, would best be evaluated by magnetic resonance imaging (MRI). The first physician implied that surgery was often needed for her symptoms. The physician's assistant scheduled her MRI and she left his office. Consulting her insurance plan benefits, Alice realized that her out-of-pocket cost for this MRI would be $1,500 since she had a

high-deductible health plan. She decided to seek
another opinion from her PCP.

After a careful history and examination, her PCP
informed her that since she had no radiation of pain,
neurological findings, or other alarming symptoms,
a conservative approach to her care with early mobi-
lization, back extension exercises, mild analgesics,
and anti-inflammatory medication was very likely
to result in improvement within a couple of weeks.
Further, the physician added that she was to return if
any worsening occurred, adding that imaging could
always be done if truly required. He explained that
her symptoms and exam placed her squarely within
evidence-based BSWQA guidelines for full recovery
using conservative care. The care plan was mutually
agreed upon.

Activated health care consumers are agents for their own
care. They may exercise this agency by choosing among
health plans, accessing and interpreting provider cost and
quality data, and understanding medical information and
treatments [155]. Patients who are more activated tend to make
more effective use of health care resources and engage in
more positive health behaviors than other patients [156], and
higher levels of patient activation have been found to be associated with better health outcomes and lower costs [157, 158].
Activated health care consumers are also more likely to seek
out health information, ask questions of providers, and be
aware of treatment guidelines [159], enabling them to participate in more effective health care decision making.

To inform and support their engagement in health care
decisions, activated patients need access to transparent data
and information about provider quality and cost of services
and treatments. Patients today are often unaware of differences in costs among health care providers because insurance
plans and benefit structures blur these cost differences. True

cost is further obscured by deductibles and co-pays. In the recent past, patients often only were exposed to the co-pay for a service, but as high-deductible health plans proliferate, often the first dollar impact to the patient is realized. As health care consumerism advances, and patients assume greater financial responsibility for their own care, the price of providers, services, and treatments is expected to become a more salient factor in health care decisions. Moreover, the question of whether a treatment or procedure is needed at all is often raised by patients today. The consumer rarely has information to know that Physician A's patients almost all receive a surgical procedure for a condition, while Physician B gets equally good results with conservative care. With proliferation of information on the Internet, alternatives are desired and being explored by patients whether or not they are offered by the health care system itself.

Reference Pricing

Reference pricing is a significant new concept illustrating how insurance companies and health care providers can make cost data more transparent to consumers (Figure 4.1) to facilitate

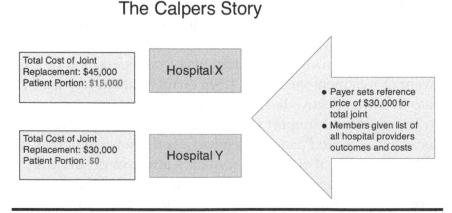

Figure 4.1   Reference pricing.

their decision making. In this example, based on actual benefit design for CalPERS beneficiaries, patient direction in their own care paths was significant.

Reference pricing provides consumers with an estimated overall cost for a procedure or treatment as well as the out-of-pocket cost to patients depending on which provider they choose. It enables consumers to weigh the cost of health care providers as well as compare their quality and thereby facilitates more informed health care decisions. The consumer knows that he or she has a certain amount of plan reimbursement that is considered reasonable for the service that is desired so he or she is motivated to spend it wisely. In this CalPERS example, if a high-cost service (Hospital X) is chosen, the consumer faces higher out-of-pocket cost. If an equally high-quality service (based on data transparency of outcomes—Hospital Y) is chosen, the reimbursement covers the entire procedure and the consumer's cost is zero. Such reference pricing has already shifted procedures from higher-cost settings to lower-cost settings [160]. The beneficiaries in this actual example rapidly chose to use equally high-quality, lower-cost facilities for their procedures. The consumers themselves literally drove a downward shift in market pricing and total costs.

Wellness, Technology, and Self-Care

As activated health care consumers take more responsibility for their own health decisions, behaviors, and outcomes, wellness, and prevention, they are assuming a more important role in care [161]. Instead of merely treating illness and disease, providers are helping patients to monitor and maintain their own health and make lifestyle choices that facilitate better health outcomes. Technology, such as wearable devices, patient portals to their own clinical records, and mobile visits, is playing a rapidly increasing role in encouraging this

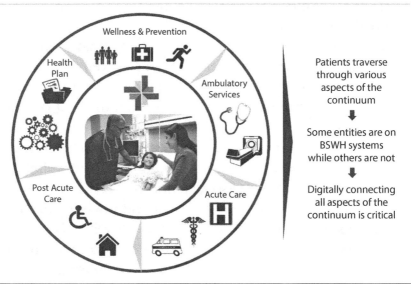

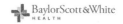

Figure 4.2 Framework for technology across the continuum of care.

enhanced patient engagement and in enabling providers
to be more patient centered across the continuum of care.
A framework for how technology can support health care
services across the care continuum is presented in Figure 4.2.
BSWH and BSWQA are deploying a set of consumer-facing
mobile health web apps, portal connections, patient information sites, and disease management resources packaged
together into an easy-to-use mobile platform, in an attempt
to provide resources from wellness through illness. Further,
BSWH linkage to insurers and transparently displaying cost
and quality information are all intended to technologically
enable a better patient experience. The digitized, activated
consumer is rapidly becoming a reality.

Mobile health (mHealth) offers many examples of how
technology can deliver lifestyle intervention support con-
veniently and inexpensively for the millions of people who
are relatively healthy, as well as those with chronic health
conditions. mHealth includes the use of portable devices
(including mobile phones, smartphones, and tablets) for

many health-related purposes, including the diagnosis, treatment, and management of a specific condition, as well as
support of general health and well-being [162]. Mobile phones,
which are almost ubiquitous (in 2013, 91% of adults in the
United States owned a mobile phone), allow the use of text
messaging to encourage wellness and healthy behaviors [163].
Patient-authorized text messages, compared to other communication channels, have the advantages of instant transmission
and low cost; they also offer economies of scale as messages
can be automated and delivered to large populations. Text
messages are also less likely to be misplaced than print
materials and, because they are asynchronous, intrude less
on daily life than phone calls [164]. With some modification,
text message–based systems can deliver the motivational
messages and monitoring and behavior change tools
previously only used in face-to-face interventions for disease
prevention and management [165]. The result is a more efficient relationship between consumers and providers.

Text messaging and other eHealth reminders, including
a variety of smartphone apps, have been found to improve
some asthma outcomes and have improved medication
compliance in patients with hypertension [164]. In another
example, electronic message reminders improved glycemic
control in patients with diabetes and reduced costs of care by
8.8% at six months, when the patient's interaction with the
system via text led to customized responses and triggered
graded alerts through a remote monitoring system with nurse
follow-up [166]. Text message–based systems can also increase
self-management capacity in some patients [164]. Patients
with a variety of chronic conditions are interested in using
mobile phone apps and text messages to assist with management, provided that privacy and security are ensured and that
out-of-pocket costs do not increase [167, 168].

The enthusiasm for mHealth is reflected in the growing volume of mHealth apps available (~100,000 in March 2013 [169]).
The consumer apps can be broadly divided into "health and

wellness" apps, including those supporting general diet and exercise programs, reference aids, symptom checkers, and similar functions, and "self-management" apps, designed to help with self-management of specific chronic conditions like hypertension, diabetes, and asthma, by allowing users to display, manage, and communicate relevant information (e.g., blood pressure and HbA1c) [170]. Many mHealth apps aggregate health data on personalized dashboards that assist consumers in making healthy lifestyle choices.

A screen shot from an mHealth app developed by BSWH for caregivers of patients with dementia is displayed in Figure 4.3 (https://itunes.apple.com/us/app/dementiaassist/id926516122?mt=8). The free app presents simple information that family members can use to care for patients with dementia, correlating gestures and facial expressions with the most effective caregiver responses.

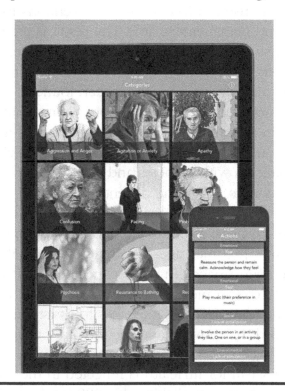

Figure 4.3   Screen shot from mHealth app for caregivers of patients with dementia.

Consumer Expectations about Access

At 7:00 p.m. on a Friday night, Laura, a mother of two young children, noticed that her 6-year-old son wasn't feeling well. He was sleepy and didn't want to eat pizza with the rest of the family, saying that his "tummy hurt." When she took his temperature, she saw that he had a low-grade fever and tucked him into bed. Over the next hour, his fever rose quickly and he became more nauseated and vomited once. Laura considered her options. The pediatrician's office had closed several hours earlier, so she wouldn't be able to take her son for an office visit. She could take him to the emergency room, but that would involve keeping him awake for most of the night for what would probably turn out to be a minor, transient illness.

Years ago, the emergency room would have been the only option for Laura, but fortunately, as a member of the BSWQA system, she had other alternatives today: a nearby ACO-connected urgent care clinic where she could check her son in via the Internet and whose staff would call her when a physician was ready to see him; an ACO-connected pharmacy retail clinic that offered after-hours access to medical care for common, acute problems; and a virtual visit to a BSWQA physician via videoconferencing on the Internet. A BSWQA member solution center, available telephonically, is in development to help Laura choose the most appropriate option from the list above.

In addition to encouraging wellness and prevention and also by enabling consumers to manage chronic conditions, mHealth and telemedicine (i.e., the use of telecommunication to provide clinical care) can improve access to care. Typically, physician office practices are open during regular business hours only on weekdays, leaving patients with fewer options for care during evenings and weekends. With telemedicine, a patient experiencing flu-like symptoms may be able to use an app to engage in videoconferencing with a provider without leaving the comfort of his or her bed, a neurologist may be able to treat a stroke patient in an isolated rural hospital, and a PCP may be able to treat a patient who has difficulty visiting a clinic (e.g., a nursing home resident or a patient with a disability). These examples illustrate how telemedicine has the potential to expand access to care across geographic regions as well as socioeconomic divides [171].

As consumers are demanding more convenient access to health care, providers are expanding mHealth and telemedicine capabilities. Approximately 42% of U.S. hospitals had adopted some form of telemedicine as of late 2012 [172], and a 2014 HIMSS Analytics survey found that 46% of more than 400 hospitals and physician practices surveyed reported using some type of telemedicine, most often videoconferencing [173]. While more widespread adoption of mHealth and telemedicine faces certain barriers, such as payer reimbursement for virtual visits and requirements for out-of-state providers to be licensed in that state in order to provide telemedicine services, both consumer demands and changes in U.S. health care policy are encouraging rapid deployment of these technologies. The proliferation of ACOs, shared financial risk among providers and payers, and the adoption of payment models that reward the meaningful use of information technology are expected to lead to the rapid expansion of mHealth and telemedicine capabilities in hospitals and physician practices across the United States [53, 174].

Retail Clinics and Access to Care

Telemedicine is just one way ACOs create opportunities for people to consult providers outside of regular business hours, and health care organizations can also improve access to care by aligning with urgent care clinics and retail clinics. Retail clinics, associated with stores such as CVS, Walgreens, and Wal-Mart, offer quick and inexpensive access to care for common health conditions, as well as screening for medical conditions such as diabetes [175]. Retail clinics are growing in prevalence; as of fall 2014, more than 1,700 were estimated to exist in the United States [176]. Many employ nurse practitioners and physician assistants who adhere strictly to evidence-based clinical practice guidelines. Retail clinics have been found to be associated with higher-quality care [177, 178] and lower consumer costs [179, 180] than emergency rooms or acute care clinics, and patients report high satisfaction with retail clinics because of their convenience and transparent pricing [181, 182]. We are finding that subsets of any patient population prefer access over relationship with physicians for selected conditions.

Many ACOs and retail clinics partner to provide high-quality, low-cost health care at locations and times that are convenient for patients. For example, Walgreens, which offers assessment, treatment, and management of asthma, diabetes, hypertension, and other chronic conditions, has joined BSWQA. With ACOs and payment models that reward strong health outcomes, Walgreens provides a needed alternative to costly, unnecessary ED visits, and ACOs benefit by referring patients to their retail partners for after-hours services [183]. Such ACO–retail clinic alliances enhance access to primary care services. As long as that care is electronically connected, the goals of a clinically integrated, high-quality, low-cost episode are easily met. Records of the care at the retail clinic can be transmitted to the ACO via an HIE. Patients, meanwhile, benefit from improved access to high-quality care at lower prices—particularly when the growth of high-deductible health care plans is making consumers more responsible for the first costs of their care [184].

Consumers Expect Patient-Centeredness

STEEEP (safe, timely, effective, efficient, equitable, patient
centered) care includes as one of its six components a
"patient-centered" approach to care. This was defined by the
IOM as care that is delivered in a way that respects patients'
needs, wants, and values [7]. Some critics observe that care in
the United States has often been designed around the needs
of the caregivers rather than those who receive care. Arcane
telephone-triage trees in physicians' offices, long waits, incon-
venient appointment times, and rushed encounters with professionals do not lead to high patient satisfaction. Physicians
and hospitals are increasingly expected to measure the satisfaction of their patients by standardized surveys, and then
to respond to those measurements by trying to continuously
improve communication, service, and response to patients'
comments. Consumerism will push the trend from these traditional shortcomings toward redesigned systems committed to
delivering the right care at the right time in the right settings
at the right cost. However, health care systems that do not
meet consumer expectations can expect competition that can
disrupt and dis-intermediate their legacy business models.

STEEEP Care in Inpatient
and Outpatient Settings

In addition to improving access to care, ACOs facilitate the
delivery of STEEEP care by encouraging stronger alignment
of quality goals and metrics across inpatient and outpatient
settings. For example, to allocate the savings that are shared
when quality health care is delivered at lower costs, ACOs
insist that their participants achieve or exceed specific quality
metrics. Physicians who partner with BSWQA must attain a
certain score across a variety of metrics related to clinical

integration within the ACO, completion of patient wellness visits, screening for conditions such as diabetes and coronary artery disease, management of chronic diseases, rate of ED visits, and rate of generic drug prescribing. Provider eligibility for BSWQA 2015 shared savings is described in more detail in Figure 4.4.

Engagement of BSWQA physicians is crucial to the success of BSWQA's clinically integrated network. Staying informed of network initiatives and monitoring individual physician performance are mandatory and considered important initial metrics for tracking progress toward clinical integration. The provider performance dashboard displayed in Figure 4.5 is an example of how this progress is measured and available to each physician through the BSWQA secure physician portal.

To demonstrate progress toward clinical integration goals, physicians are required to complete the clinical integration criteria as outlined in the shared savings distribution model in Figure 4.4. Failure to attain this measure eliminates a physician from any shared savings percentages as described below.

70% for Primary Care

Seventy percent of the shared savings is allocated to PCMH physicians and is distributed as follows: 50% based on BSWQA Medicare Advantage (contract measures) *and* commercial contracts (contract measures), both calculated by patient panel size, and 20% for community (global measures). One might ask, "Why is 70% of a shared savings pool allocated to primary care?" Although both primary care and specialist practices manage the overall health of their patients, a significant amount of time spent caring for and managing high-risk patients falls to the PCP. While this time spent in disease management is critical, much of it, such as care between visits, is not reimbursed. The ACO is asking PCPs to truly function as "comprehensivists," giving continuing care above

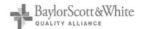

ACHIEVING YOUR
2015 SHARED SAVINGS

Physicians must be participating providers with BSWQA health plan contracts in order to be eligible for shared savings

Clinical Integration

Clinical Integration MUST be completed by ALL physicians in order to participate in ANY shared savings

▸ **Patient Satisfaction Survey** - *Attest to surveying patients with a government approved vendor • Applies to those specialties reporting patient satisfaction*

▸ **Attend at least 1 Pod Meeting** (*Regional Town Hall*)
▸ **Accumulate 10 clinical integration points as follows:**
  • 1 point = One website login per month
  • 5 points = BSWQA assigned eCME
  • 5 points = One MRA training

Primary Care

PCMH Application Submission is required to receive shared savings with PCMH recognition level calculated on a pro rata basis:
  • Level 1 = 50%
  • Lavel 2 = 80%
  • Level 3 = 100%

Contract Measures (50%)
▸ **Medicare Advantage**
  • Wellness Visit Completion - 75%
  • Diabetic population (HbA1c) - 80%
  • Chronic disease appointment - 70%
▸ **Commercial Contract**
  • Diabetic population (HbA1c) - 93%
  • Diabetes (Nephropathy screening) - 93%
  • CAD patients LDL-C screening - TBD

Community Measures (20%)
▸ **ED Visits/1,000**
▸ **Generic Prescribing Rate**

Specialty Care

BSWQA Measures (*measures which apply globally to the contract*)
▸ **Efficiency Measures**
  • ED Visits/1,000
  • Generic Prescribing Rate

For a complete description of the BSWQA shared savings distribution model, we invite you to read the shared savings white paper located at members.baylorqualityalliance.com/shared-savings

Figure 4.4   Baylor Scott & White Quality Alliance 2015 requirements for provider participation in shared savings.

Provider Performance Dashboard

Family Medicine

BaylorScott&White QUALITY ALLIANCE

2015 Shared Savings Requirements

Data for physicians without EHR connectivity (i.e. claims data only) is delayed 60-90 days because of the time it takes for claim processing.

Metric Name	Current Period	Prior Period	Target	Percentile
Clinical Integration Pool: Earn 10 points for the year; Monthly Website Login: 1 point; BSWQA Assigned eCME: 5 points; MRA Training: 5 points	20.0% 2 of 10 01/01/2015 to 05/31/2015	10.0% 1 of 10 01/01/2015 to 04/30/2015	10	58th
Clinical Integration: Patient Satisfaction Surveys; Goal: Survey patients using an approved CG-CAHPS vendor	100.0% 1 of 1 01/01/2015 to 05/31/2015	100.0% 1 of 1 01/01/2015 to 04/30/2015	1	99th
Clinical Integration: Attend POD Meeting; Goal: Attend 1 meeting	0.0% 0 of 1 01/01/2015 to 05/31/2015	0.0% 0 of 1 01/01/2015 to 04/30/2015	1	84th
Primary Care: PCMH Application Submitted to NCQA; Goal: Recognition of Patient Centered Medical Home	100.0% 1 of 1 01/01/2015 to 05/31/2015	100.0% 1 of 1 01/01/2015 to 04/30/2015	1	99th
Primary Care: Generic prescribing rate; Goal: 86.7%	84.0% 9390 of 11184 01/01/2014 to 01/31/2015	84.0% 96453 of 114881 01/01/2014 to 12/31/2014	86.7	99th

Service

Metric Name	Current Period	Prior Period	Target	Percentile

Text in blue links to a report with additional detail.
Additional inpatient service line reports are available by clicking here.

Quality

Data is from EHRs and billing where BSWQA has established connectivity and claims data from all BSWQA contracts. Data for physicians without EHR connectivity (i.e. claims data only) is delayed 60-90 days because of the time it takes for claim processing.

Metric Name	Current Period	Prior Period	Target	Percentile
Influenza vaccination: 2014-15 flu season (6mos and older)	37.0% 424 of 1146 05/01/2014 to 04/30/2015	37.3% 431 of 1156 04/01/2014 to 03/31/2015		31st
Pneumonia vaccination (ever) (age 65+)	81.5% 97 of 119 05/01/2014 to 04/30/2015	81.1% 99 of 122 04/01/2014 to 03/31/2015		26th
DM: LDL < 100 or >= 100 with documented plan incl statin prescription (18-75yo)	81.9% 59 of 72 05/01/2014 to 04/30/2015	79.7% 59 of 74 04/01/2014 to 03/31/2015		14th
Wellness visit completion (65yo+)	5.0% 6 of 119 05/01/2014 to 04/30/2015	5.0% 6 of 121 04/01/2014 to 03/31/2015		11th
HTN: Blood pressure in control (140090 for 18-59y/o, 150/90 for 65+)	78.1% 210 of 269 05/01/2014 to 04/30/2015	77.6% 201 of 259 04/01/2014 to 03/31/2015		30th

Link to I-TPN Provider Dashboard (For all your HTPN Financial, Quality, and Service data) NOTE: *This link will only work on the Baylor Network*

Utilization Efficiency

Metric Name	Current Period	Prior Period	Target	Percentile
Generic Prescribing Rate	73.7% YTD through: 11/23/2014	69.3% 1/1/2013 to 12/31/2013		

Figure 4.5 Sample provider performance dashboard.

and beyond visits. The long-term success of the BSWQA is
heavily dependent on improving population health management. Most cost savings realized by any payer will be generated within the PCMH pool, and thus PCMH-recognized
physicians should be accorded a higher proportionate share
of any shared savings. Physicians who attain Level 3 NCQA
PCMH recognition receive their full share from this segment
of the pool, physicians who attain Level 2 recognition receive
an 80% share, and Level 1–recognized physicians receive
a 20% share.

20% for Specialty Care

Twenty percent of the shared savings is allocated to specialist
physicians and distributed pro rata. Specialist physicians
play a vital role in ensuring appropriate access to and use
of other specialty services by patients and their PCPs. They
play a large role in helping patients remain in network.
Coordination of care among the specialist, PCP, and other
providers is expected. Effective, timely communication
between specialists and referring PCPs will increase in
importance, both to avoid duplication and to guide the PCPs
in ideal patient treatment. The specialist must also provide
appropriate care in a cost-effective manner, and that contribution will be rewarded.

10% for All Physicians

Recognizing that all physician members of BSWQA have roles
to play, and because of the desire to engage those physicians
who even see a very low number of patients, the board of
BSWQA decided to allocate the remaining 10% of the shared
savings pool to all physician members. Even though the
amount per physician is low, it underscores the collaborative
nature of membership in the alliance.

Shared Savings and the Patient Experience of Care

Provider participation in shared savings enhances the experience of care in several important ways. First, providers are required to demonstrate evidence of efforts to clinically integrate with the BSWQA through specific patient-centered activities such as the administration of patient satisfaction surveys. Second, the BSWQA focus on wellness visits (described in more detail in Chapter 5), and chronic disease screening and management improves patients' experience of care by facilitating a connection between patients and providers even in times of wellness, and by helping patients to become more empowered to prevent and manage chronic health conditions. All physician members of BSWQA are required to access the secure member website eight of 12 months and to attend a regional POD meeting annually. The POD meetings are growing in popularity due to the opportunity for specialists and PCP interaction plus the mutual review of performance data. Finally, to be eligible for shared savings, providers need to demonstrate a commitment to preventing ED visits, a goal that is achieved both by improving patients' ability to manage their own health and by ensuring that care is available to patients at times and locations that are convenient for them. All of these actions are integral to enhancing patients' experience of care.

Role of Hospitals in Population Health

Hospitals play an important role in achieving the Triple Aim, particularly in improving the health of populations [1]. Hospitals are especially well positioned to facilitate the delivery of value-based care via the avoidance of adverse events and readmissions—goals that are aligned with STEEEP aims. The Hospital-Acquired Condition Reduction Program, formalized in the ACA, establishes a reduction in payment for hospitals that fall within the worst-performing quartile on measures of adverse events occurring during hospital stays, such as pressure ulcers, pulmonary embolisms, and health care–associated conditions [185, 186]. Similarly, the Readmissions Reduction Program reduces payment for facilities with high rates of rehospitalization within 30 days of discharge for heart failure, pneumonia, and acute myocardial infarction [187]. As noted previously, the financial penalties to institutions performing poorly are growing in magnitude (see Figure 2.6). CMS is seeking *accountability* for performance and is willing to use its payment authority to achieve it. These programs help to ensure that hospitals are paid for acute care services based on quality of care rather than quantity of services provided and contribute to improved population health by preventing patients from experiencing frequent, costly readmissions. Reduction of adverse events and hospital readmissions also enhances the achievement of STEEEP care, especially patient safety, clinical effectiveness, and care efficiency. Preventing hospital admissions—a goal that is facilitated by improving patients' ability to manage their own health and by ensuring that care is available to patients at times and locations that are convenient for them—is also important to improving the patient experience of care.

Integration between Hospital Care and Ambulatory Care

Improving the health of populations requires integration of goals, initiatives, and metrics between hospital care and ambulatory care settings. Many efforts to reduce hospital readmission, for example, focus on the transition from hospital to home or to a post–acute care facility, such as a long-term acute care facility (LTAC) or skilled nursing facility (SNF). Care transitions can be confusing for patients and are often associated with poor care coordination among providers and lack of effective postdischarge planning [6]. To address these issues, a variety of transitional care programs have been developed and shown to reduce readmission rates, ED use, and hospital length of stay, improving the quality and reducing the cost of care [188–191]. These include improved patient education and postdischarge nurse telemonitoring, efforts to improve medication instructions at discharge, and both physician- and nurse-led postdischarge house calls. The proliferation of such initiatives highlights the importance of care coordination between hospital and ambulatory settings in improving the quality and efficiency of care and enhancing the health of populations. Such initiatives improve the patient experience of care through enhanced patient satisfaction, decreases in hospital readmission as patients achieve a better understanding of their diagnoses and medication instructions, and the assurance of an ongoing connection between patients and providers through telemonitoring or house calls.

BSWQA has invested significantly in an ambulatory care coordination infrastructure. Because of the necessity of coordinating care for patients most at risk (complex patients, transitional patients, and patients predicted to be at high risk), a multilayered coordination of care structure was developed. Nurse care managers work with the most complex patients, medical assistants coordinate visits and close care gaps, and social workers intervene in resolving barriers to care as well as certain behavioral situations. More detail is found in Chapter 5.

Since care coordination depends on the existence of a network of health care providers and facilities that are committed to delivering high-quality, patient-centered care, BSWQA members include a number of SNFs and LTACs as well as selected home health agencies. Each was selected based upon known quality criteria, and each signed a participation agreement to connect electronically, follow discharge care protocols, complete advanced directives, report on known post–acute care criteria such as falls and infections, and work closely with the ACO to prevent unnecessary rehospitalization.

Hospital and ambulatory care settings can also improve care integration through the use of information technology, particularly HIEs. HIEs allow the electronic movement of clinical information across different health information systems while maintaining the integrity of the information being exchanged [76]. The BSWQA HIE provides connectivity among the EHRs of a variety of affiliated entities, including post–acute care facilities, hospitals, and physicians, assimilating a robust clinical record from relevant data from these sources. Additionally, the HIE provides a "community view" of a patient's record to any provider at the point of care, enabling real-time access to a patient's medical history and other pertinent clinical information. (See Chapter 5 for a more detailed description of the BSWQA HIE.) HIEs help to consolidate patient information across care settings and episodes of care, facilitating data integration, providing a more complete picture of a patient's entire care trajectory, and driving improved care in accordance with STEEEP aims. The integration of care fostered by HIEs improves the patient experience of care by enabling a more seamless patient journey through the health care system and ensuring that each provider can make treatment decisions that are informed by patient data and by health records collected during previous care encounters. BSWQA postacute care members, hospitals, and physicians all hold themselves *accountable* to share data for care and data for performance, and to access that data to prevent redundancy and improve outcomes.

Chapter 5

Population Health

Main Points for Chapter

This chapter includes a discussion of:

- How accountable care organizations define and care for populations of patients
- Primary care and the patient-centered medical home
- The role of nurse care coordinators in population health
- The importance of information technology, including electronic health records, health information exchanges, and analytic reports in driving coordinated care
- The role of wellness programs in promoting accountable care

Until the passage of the ACA [14] and the development of the Triple Aim framework [1], there had been no directive for physicians and health care systems to manage the health of any population (some of whose members may not even be actively engaged in care at the moment) and there had been no mandate to seriously control costs. In a fee-for-service world, the system and the physicians are usually only paid for visits and procedures. With the arrival of the Triple Aim, BSWH and other health systems across the nation are being challenged to broaden their focus beyond improving the quality of care they deliver to patients to now include the two additional dimensions of the Triple Aim: improving the health of populations and reducing the per capita cost of health care.

In most health settings today, no one is accountable for all three dimensions of the IHI Triple Aim. Population health strategies promote the clinical integration of various health systems to effectively and efficiently manage the care of the entire population, particularly the top 5% of chronically ill patients who are considered high risk and whose care consumes 50% of health care costs [192]. Keeping these patients well and in control of their conditions is considered to be one of the most effective means for reducing health care costs in this country. Managing the care for these highest-risk patients—those diagnosed with chronic disease such as diabetes, heart failure, COPD, cancer, and asthma—and assisting them to more effectively manage their conditions, has proven to reduce negative population health outcomes such as avoidable ED utilization, preventable hospital admissions, and 30-day readmissions, and to reduce overall costs [190].

The starting point for any health system committing to a population health strategy is to agree upon a strategy for population health that is relevant to the organization and then embark on creating an investment plan for building a uniform infrastructure. At the inception of the BSWQA, a framework was developed that began to approach population health from four key areas (Figure 5.1): redefining the entry point (i.e., PCMH), aligning with willing specialists and hospitals, building population health tools and infrastructure, and creating financial payment changes to reward population health. This framework recognizes that fee-for-service payments alone do not sufficiently fund *accountability* for population health improvement, and has proven valid as a model since the inception of BSWQA.

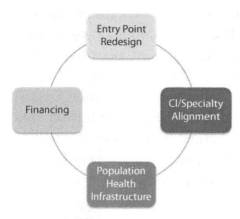

Entry Point Redesign:
Primary Care strength, PCP, PCMH, referral leverage, access & capacity challenge

Care Integration/Specialty Alignment:
Large scale physician partnering, private practice challenge, BSWH hospital strength, HIT deployment

Population Health Infrastructure:
Disproportionate resource allocation, quality & cost reduction mandate

Financing:
Texas Collaborative, new payment models, product/benefit design & data control

Figure 5.1 Four key approaches to improving population health.

The formation of BSWQA necessitated answering questions like "What does population health mean for us?" For physicians, the frequent question of "What's in this for me?" had to be addressed. Although some financial rewards were anticipated in shared savings for physicians, they had to grasp the greater good of the ACO strategy. Empowering staff at all levels and linking organizational goals to population health were important components of building the infrastructure, which also entailed designing the systems to meet comprehensive patient needs and prioritizing costly investments such as information technology, care coordination, and data analytics [193]. BSWQA is committed to the advancement of population health by improving quality of care, positively impacting health outcomes, and reducing preventable health care costs for those patients with chronic conditions at the highest level of risk.

Baylor Scott & White Quality Alliance Population Health Infrastructure

BSWQA began designing its population health infrastructure around the enhancement and deployment of already well-established HTPN initiatives centered on care management and clinical integration. These included adult preventive health services, chronic disease management, network-wide implementation of an EHR, and the redesign of primary care practices as PCMHs. BSWQA's road map to population health stems from HTPN's long and successful history of tracking and monitoring the health status of patient populations through its chronic disease registries and clinical management program that promotes evidence-based management of care [33, 35, 194, 195].

Practicing evidence-based medicine requires physician orders. Standardizing common orders around evidence becomes a very important organizational priority. Starting from HTPN's catalog of evidence-based protocols, BSWQA physicians have continued the development of both primary care protocols and more than 110 specialty-originated, board-approved protocols that are being utilized in BSWQA practices to standardize care and manage chronically ill patients diagnosed with diabetes, heart failure, COPD, and asthma. These protocols are distributed over the BSWQA member portal and tracked for performance, which is fed back to practitioners. In addition, HTPN's high performance in adult preventive health services has paved the way for great progress in altering health behaviors and changing risk profiles for high-risk patients while simultaneously promoting wellness. The spread of these two programs as well as the PCMH efforts initiated throughout the BSWQA network, coupled with investments in care coordination and a suite of data analytic solutions, has served as the catalyst for BSWQA's population health infrastructure and the development of new care models focused on clinical integration and accountability. Assembling all of the components of population health has been a detailed and strenuous organizational accomplishment. Six of the key elements are pictured in Figure 5.2 and amplified in the discussion that follows.

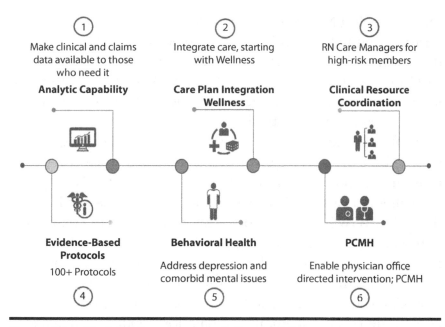

Figure 5.2 Six initiatives for population health management.

Patient-Centered Medical Home

The PCMH provides an evidence-based, solid foundation for accessible, high-quality, patient-centered care and is considered a proven effective model for influencing and achieving the broader elements of the Triple Aim initiative. Many industry experts agree that the most effective approach for reorienting the health care system to efficiently and effectively manage growing patient panels with complex medical conditions is to initiate the PCMH model of care in tandem with an accountable care infrastructure and incentives (i.e., shared savings) to facilitate collaboration across the care continuum [17, 147]. Primary care is the fundamental base, but the ACO components must include specialty physicians, hospitals, post–acute care, retail care sites, and other health care stakeholders.

Early development of the PCMH model began with the redesign of BSWQA's primary care practices within HTPN. The existing attainment of the status of Level 3, the highest level NCQA PCMH certification, is the foundation for BSWQA's more than 100 NCQA-recognized PCMH primary care sites representing more than 500 providers located throughout the north and central Texas regions of the network. These NCQA-recognized PCMH care sites include clinics focused on family medicine, internal medicine, and pediatrics, as well as senior centers and charity clinics.

To further expand the network's NCQA PCMH recognition efforts, BSWQA offers administrative and field support for those independent primary care practices pursuing NCQA recognition as a PCMH. The application process is facilitated through a BSWQA field support staff and physician champions at the practice level, providing physician-to-physician com- munication and coaching for engagement and attainment of NCQA PCMH status. NCQA's list of elements considered essential to the PCMH include patient-centered appointment access, the practice team, use of data for population manage- ment, care planning and self-care support, referral tracking and follow-up, and implementation of continuous quality improvement (Figure 5.3) [196]. Because of Stark limitations

---

The Standards

The PCMH 2014 program's six standards align with the core components of primary care.

1. PCMH 1: Patient-Centered Access.
2. PCMH 2: Team-Based Care.
3. PCMH 3: Population Health Management.
4. PCMH 4: Care Management and Support.
5. PCMH 5: Care Coordination and Care Transitions.
6. PCMH 6: Performance Measurement and Quality Improvement.

The Must-Pass Elements

Six must-pass elements are considered essential to the patient-centered medical home, and are required for practices at all recognition levels. Practices must achieve a score of 50% or higher on must-pass elements:

1. PCMH 1, Element A: Patient-Centered Appointment Access.
2. PCMH 2, Element D: The Practice Team.
3. PCMH 3, Element D: Use Data for Population Management.
4. PCMH 4, Element B: Care Planning and Self-Care Support.
5. PCMH 5, Element B: Referral Tracking and Follow-Up.
6. PCMH 6, Element D: Implement Continuous Quality Improvement.

Figure 5.3 National Committee on Quality Assurance patient-centered medical home standards.

(Chapter 3), the level of support for independent physicians is more informative than hands-on.

With solid experience in adult preventive health services and disease management established, guidelines for coordinating care are already largely in place. Adherence to PCMH guidelines is monitored through weekly tracking reports submitted to the PCMH department. PCMH criteria for specialists are just emerging from NCQA. In its principles for reward distribution, BSWQA awards highest potential payments to primary care practices with Level 3 certification, less to Levels 1 and 2, and none to practices that have not begun NCQA certification (see Chapter 4 for more details about shared savings).

BSWQA's PCMH model was further designed by enhancing existing preventive health services and disease management infrastructures. Resources such as registered nurse care coordination, advanced practice providers, and decision support tools were augmented to achieve fundamental PCMH components of comprehensive, patient-centered, team-based, and coordinated care as well as accessibility and quality [197]. Patients in a BSWQA medical home are paired with a dedicated PCP who agrees to be held *accountable* for providing comprehensive, quality care in a coordinated manner. The PCP guides a care team involving advanced practice providers, nurse care managers, health coordinators, and social workers to assist patients with ED and inpatient and postdischarge transitions, monitor chronic conditions, identify gaps in care, manage psychosocially complex cases, and promote wellness. Care is coordinated across multiple care settings that may include hospitals, specialists, post–acute care, and community services.

Transitioning BSWQA practices to NCQA-recognized PCMHs has revitalized primary care delivery and prompted a renewed focus on primary care and the important role it plays in shifting from volume to value. BSWQA's PCMH strategy has demonstrated positive results for improving quality and safety for patients, while simultaneously creating a foundation for care coordination and population health management throughout the BSWQA network of clinics. Through PCMH initiatives, BSWQA has incorporated key elements of managing patient populations such as evidence-based medicine, care standards, a team approach to care, expanded access, coordinated care, community care, patient education, social work, preventive health, wellness, and disease management.

While one important cornerstone of the PCMH model is to focus on meeting the needs and preferences of patients, another is payment reform that improves reimbursement to primary care practices and rewards the degree to which the PCP meets performance thresholds in the comprehensive role of care manager. The role of the ACO in complementing the PCMH model with infrastructure and incentives (i.e., shared savings) becomes essential as PCPs are challenged to implement the requirements of health care reform and its effect on their economic status. Primary care physicians are trained to comprehensively manage chronic disease as well as acute care. However, because fee-for-service payments in the primary care setting reward episodic, simple care better than complex care, new payment incentives will be needed. At the time of this publication, further alternative payment models for primary care are under consideration. These models being considered include partial and full capitation to recognize that the work of a "comprehensivist" PCP includes significant efforts over and beyond office visits. All such models should enhance the effective delivery of population health.

In order to remain competitive in patient-centered care and continue on BSWQA's quest to close care gaps, engage in population health management, and deliver value-based care to patients, BSWQA continues to submit applications on behalf of new and existing practices to meet the current NCQA standards for a PCMH.

BSWQA Specialists and Care Protocols Complete the Total Care Experience

The integration of BSWQA specialists within the medical home model advances the routine patient encounter to a more comprehensive, *total care experience*. BSWQA specialty care physicians represent a broad spectrum of services that includes allergy, breast surgery, cancer care, cardiology, critical care, dermatology, endocrinology, gastroenterology, general surgery, geriatrics, gynecology, hepatology, neuro-oncology, neurology, neurosurgery, obstetrics, orthopedic surgery, orthopedic trauma, otolaryngology, pulmonology, radiology, radiosurgery, rheumatology, thoracic surgery, transplant surgery, urogynecology, urology, and wound care. BSWQA's network of specialty services facilitates PCPs having ample opportunities for specialty alignment resulting in better communication, advanced treatment options, and a higher level of coordinated care for their patients. Specialty and primary care alignment also nurtures PCMH recruitment and sustainability while simultaneously improving quality and lowering costs through better management of patient populations. Specialists and PCPs collaborate on all evidence-based care protocols and are linked electronically by EHR and HIE technology. PCPs and specialists meet in regional PODs semiannually and jointly view their disease management and efficiency reports.

Care Coordination

The complexity of care of patients today has never been higher. A hospital stay may involve dozens of non-physician providers, multiple physicians, and result in complicated, often confusing discharge and transactional instructions. In a recent example, an elderly patient was discharged on six medications. The following day, a BSWQA RN care manager contacted the patient, only to learn that she was indeed taking the six medications—plus twenty-nine other medications that she had. A pharmacist was promptly sent to her home by a BSWQA care manager, the medications were reconciled, and a likely disaster was averted.

According to the National Quality Forum, "Care coordination is a function that helps ensure that the patient's needs and preferences for health services and information sharing between practitioners, and between sites, are met over time. Coordination maximizes the value of services delivered to patients by facilitating beneficial, efficient, safe, and high-quality patient experiences and improved health care outcomes" [198]. BSWQA supports coordination of care through a significant investment in staff and programs. In addition to coordination of care that is practice-based within PCMHs, BSWQA has created a centralized care coordination department consisting of registered nurse care managers, health coordinators, and social workers.

The care coordination function reports to the chief medical officer of BSWQA. Its protocols are governed by the Best Care/Clinical Integration Committee (see Chapter 3 for more details). Care coordination outcome and process metrics are routinely evaluated by the chief medical officer and the BSWQA Care Coordination Committee. Opportunities are identified and acted upon utilizing the process improvement plan, do, check, act cycle commonly enacted through BSWH's process improvement tools, and *accountable* performance is enhanced by medical directors, physician champions, and chairs of specialty subcommittees.

Care Coordination Workflow

Centralized care coordination supports complex care management for the highest-risk patients who have been identified through risk stratification and predictive modeling and for high-risk transitions of care from the hospital to home. Physicians may additionally request care coordination for patients needing help beyond the practice's resources. Considered by patients to be an extension of the BSWQA physician's practice, the nurse care manager provides a valuable response to the PCP team that does not typically exist in the fee-for-service world. BSWQA care coordination professionals augment the health management of the physician's highest-risk patients and are requested by patients as a valuable extender of their physician's team. They help to ensure that medications are regularly reconciled. The patient's care plan is devised and driven by the PCP. The responsibilities of the BSWQA care coordination team are to reinforce the physician's care plan and assist the patient in attaining compliance. Through shared decision making and motivational interviewing approaches, the nurse care manager works with the patient and the physician to deliver the tools patients need to reach their individual health goals. Integral to the model is ongoing communication with the patient's PCP, as well as collaboration by care coordination staff with specialists and other sites of care. A flowchart for care coordination is presented in Figure 5.4.

The BSWQA care coordination team consists of nurse care managers (one for every 250 patients with private insurance and one for every 150 Medicare and Medicare Advantage patients), social workers (for patients needing higher levels of psychological or sociological support), and certified medical assistant (CMA) health coordinators

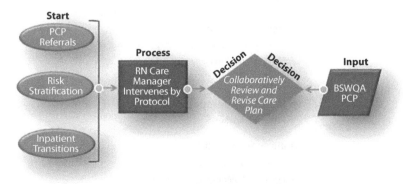

Figure 5.4   Care coordination workflow.

(one for every 1,000 patients with private insurance and one for every 500 Medicare and Medicare Advantage patients). CMA health coordinators take responsibility for tasks that do not require nurse expertise (e.g., scheduling appointments and identifying and closing care gaps through the data systems). Each PCP is assigned a team member in each of these categories to whom they can refer patients, and patients are assigned support according to their risk category: the 5% with the highest risk are assigned a nurse care manager, and the next 15% are assigned a health coordinator. When the initial assessment conducted by the care manager or health coordinator indicates that the patient is in need of resources to address the social determinants of health, such as housing or transportation to access medical care, or behavioral health issues, the patient may be referred to the social worker, who conducts an in-depth assessment and can help link the patient to organizations that assist with the needed resources.

The areas of care that care coordination targets are wellness, prevention, and care transitions (specifically, primary care follow-up after an ED visit or hospital admission), as well as evidence-based disease management for patients with complex chronic diseases. Figure 5.5 shows the functions each team member performs.

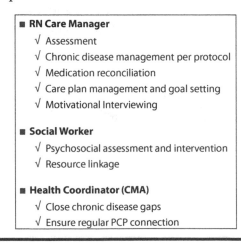

■ RN Care Manager
√ Assessment
√ Chronic disease management per protocol
√ Medication reconciliation
√ Care plan management and goal setting
√ Motivational Interviewing

■ Social Worker
√ Psychosocial assessment and intervention
√ Resource linkage

■ Health Coordinator (CMA)
√ Close chronic disease gaps
√ Ensure regular PCP connection

Figure 5.5   Roles of care coordination team members.

Preliminary results from the use of care coordination demonstrate substantial success, with 74% of the high- or rising-risk population having been engaged, and outcomes data showing a decrease in readmission rates among Medicare Advantage patients from 16% to 11% with the implementation of care coordination. Comparisons of intermediate clinical outcome measures for chronic conditions (such as the proportion of patients meeting the recommended thresholds for HbA1c, LDL cholesterol, and blood pressure) between patients who have and have not engaged with the care coordinators also show better performance with care coordination. Physicians report finding their care coordinators invaluable for meeting the needs of complex patients, particularly as patients are able to access these resources between physician office visits.

Currently, most contact between the care coordinators and patients occurs via telephone, and between care coordinators and clinical providers via the EHR or, when an urgent matter arises, by telephone. Work is underway to add text, email, and web portal communication options for patients, and in the future, care coordinators may be embedded in practices, as a critical volume of contracted patients is acquired in the practice. Care coordinators also visit SNF units to follow network patients.

> Fred, age 73, had not seen a PCP in more than three years. Upon enrollment with BSQWA, he was identified as a high-risk patient and was immediately contacted by a nurse care manager. The nurse care manager met telephonically with Fred and asked him about his recent medical history and current medications. She discovered that the symptoms of Fred's chronic health conditions, which included diabetes and heart failure, had worsened during the last several years and that he had seen several specialists since his last visit to his PCP. He had been prescribed six different medications to help control his conditions.

Because Fred's care for the past several years had
not been coordinated through the PCP's office, two
of the specialists, not knowing Fred's entire medical history, had each prescribed Fred a different beta
blocker. After conferring immediately by phone with
the PCP, the nurse directed Fred to immediately stop
one of the beta blockers. An urgent appointment was
made to engage Fred with his PCP in a PCMH. He
was confused about the role of each of his medications and needed help from the PCP, the nurse care
manager, his specialists, and the care coordination
team to sort out the error, and therefore likely avoid
a major drug-related adverse event.

Motivational Interviewing

Motivational interviewing is a technique used by nurse care
managers to ask open-ended questions of patients about
their personal goals in respect to their health. Example questions include "What health goals are you trying to achieve?"
"How are you feeling?" and "What did you hear your doctor
say?" A typical BSWQA nurse care manager-to-patient conver-
sation allows the patient to self-determine his or her health
status, wishes, and goals. If we take Fred's health scenario into
consideration, he may have had a nurse care manager call him
after his eventual follow-up visit to his PCP that would have
proceeded as follows: "I see that you saw Dr. Jones two days
ago and at that time the two of you discussed your diabetes.
Can you tell me what your understanding of that discussion
was?" Fred might reply, "Well, Dr. Jones said I am doing
really well." To which the nurse care manager might respond,
"That's great, I see from your chart that there were some
medication changes while you were there. What is your understanding of why those medications were changed?" Fred might
reply, "I can't remember why my medications were changed.
Can you review with me what I am supposed to do?"

Open-ended questions like these help patients to come to the realization on their own that they may not have a clear understanding of their care plan or instructions after all. Using motivational interviewing techniques reinforces patient autonomy and self-determination, which improves the odds of patient compliance with the treatment plan [199]. Engaging patients in this way provides them with a feeling of empowerment and confidence in their ability to control their conditions, in contrast to the more traditional, paternalistic approach to medicine, which often amounts to an assumption that "if patients are told what to do, our professional work is done. The rest is 'up to the patient.'" We know today that such reasoning is obsolete.

In addition to the nurse care managers who skillfully assist in transitional care and complex disease management, BSWQA health coordinators monitor ED and inpatient transitions and complete a protocol-driven patient outreach following those encounters. The non-nurse health coordinators work with the health care team, focusing primarily on promoting wellness and closing gaps in care for adult preventive care services. They also monitor patients with chronic diseases and facilitate follow-up appointments with their PCPs.

Supplementing the nurse care managers and health coordinators are licensed social workers. Hospital readmissions are often due in part to social factors such as socioeconomic status, education, and lack of social support [200]. Patients may be admitted to the hospital because certain social barriers create an inability to adhere to treatment plans devised by their physician or the patient simply lacks the coping mechanisms necessary to overcome barriers [201]. The job of the social worker is to identify multiple potential barriers a patient may encounter while carrying out the treatment plan prescribed by the doctor, such as inability to afford medications or lack of transportation to a pharmacy to get prescriptions filled. The skill of the social worker to perform a psychosocial assessment on the patient, discover the root of the problem, and then connect the patient to the appropriate resources (community or otherwise) can assist greatly in resolving the issue.

An initial psychosocial assessment conducted on a patient involves (1) determining the patient's level of help at home, (2) uncovering any behavioral issues such as depression or other mental illness, and (3) uncovering financial barriers that may hinder the patient's ability to pay for medication or housing. Any barriers to care identified are addressed through the care coordination department, attempts are made to overcome those barriers, and then this information is communicated to the physician through the EHR.

The most frail, elderly, high-risk inpatients with a diagnosis of heart failure, pneumonia, or COPD who are discharged to their home may receive additional services from a multidisciplinary transitional care team consisting of an advanced practice nurse, a nurse, a pharmacist, and a social worker for 30 to 90 days. The services include follow-up calls from a transitional care registered nurse, remote monitoring, and home visits. The pharmacist reviews the patient's discharge medication list and assesses the possibility of reducing the number of medications as well as the potential for drug-to-drug or drug-to-food interactions [202]. Cognitive disorders in this population are often identified, necessitating deeper engagement of family caregivers.

Care Coordinator "Hot List" Workflows

Focusing expensive nursing resources requires prioritization and intentionality. Care coordination workflows have been established and deployed to review a population hot list and schedule the appropriate clinic visit needed according to the clinic's scheduling preferences directly in the practice management system. These visits include both wellness and disease management visits across all populations—commercial, traditional Medicare, and Medicare Advantage. Lists of patients who have not had wellness visits, who have gaps in preventive services, or who have not had regular diabetes or hypertensive visits are presented to the care coordination team, who reach out to patients and counsel or schedule visits—closing these care gaps.

Transitional Care

In order to be effective, both system and individual *accountability* are needed. The BSWQA transitional care model particularly targets the sickest elderly patients (65 years or older) such as those who have been diagnosed with heart failure. The primary features of BSWQA's transitional care model consist of assigning a nurse practitioner (with physician oversight) as the case manager or leader of care and include dedicated follow-up, in-home care for all heart failure patients upon discharge. Nurse practitioners work in collaboration with BSWH physicians and staff to manage the discharge planning process of patients with heart failure. The patient and the dedicated nurse practitioner, together, review heart failure information packets and set mutually agreed upon goals for postdischarge treatment plans. Follow-up care is provided through home visits, phone calls, and remote monitoring. The goal for the nurse practitioner is to establish a rapport with the patient and build a relationship based on trust with the patient, family, physicians, and hospital staff.

Initial nurse practitioner contact occurs within 24 to 72 hours of a heart failure patient's hospital admission. Upon receipt of discharge orders by the patient, the nurse performs the following transitional care interventions:

■ Assesses caregiver needs and coordinated discharge plans with patient and family
■ Assists patient with understanding and managing heart failure symptoms, including dietary salt restrictions and daily weights, and reporting abnormal weight gain or shortness of breath

■ Provides extensive education on plan of care, including medication management
■ Facilitates communication and transition to the residential home, home with home health care, or assisted living facility
■ Enables access to dedicated nurse practitioner seven days per week for home visits or follow-up phone calls
■ Performs at least eight nurse practitioner home visits following patient's hospital discharge, with geriatrician oversight

Transitional care nurse practitioners are certified in heart failure through the American Association of Heart Failure Nurses and are encouraged to regularly attend continuing education courses related to heart failure. In their role as transitional care nurses, they have significant *accountability*. Weekly case conferences are held between the lead nurse practitioner and his or her team to discuss protocol adherence and difficult cases. These meetings rely heavily on team input so that early warnings of deterioration can be caught and corrected if possible. If readmissions occur, they are reviewed to identify any possible protocol failures.

The transitional care model utilized by BSWQA differs slightly from the industry-wide transitional care model pioneered by Naylor et al. [189] in that BSWQA nurses use "prudent prescriptive authority" as they teach self-care management skills to patients and caregivers. If medications need to be prescribed, acute illnesses need to be treated, or labs need to be checked, the nurse practitioner can provide these services. Nurses are required to report any services provided to the patient's geriatric PCP or primary cardiologist and utilize a shared EHR as well as the HIE [191, 202].

Data Analytics

Good data are fundamental for ACOs to function [58]. All too often, high-risk, chronically ill patients follow a path of costly diagnostics, treatments in acute care settings, discharge with unclear instructions for follow-up, and then eventual readmission for the same disease within 30 days of discharge. Data-derived analytic tools provide the means for transforming clinical data into meaningful, actionable information resulting in effective and efficient population health interventions producing better outcomes. These tools allow for the aggregation of multiple clinical data sources such as inpatient and outpatient EHRs, inpatient and outpatient practice management systems, and claims downloads from each contracted payer group, resulting in a longitudinal view of patients as well as population-based reporting that can be used for evaluating and optimizing the care delivered and the process by which it is delivered. Good data identify patients whose care may need additional resources (excessive ED visits) or something as simple as gaps in care (lack of a flu shot or a mammogram).

With access to and understanding of actionable data it is possible to create, deploy, and measure the effects of evidence-based disease protocols, order sets, clinical guidelines, barriers to goals, health care maintenance reminders, and many other initiatives that "intelligently" target patient-specific clinical needs based upon patient-specific relevant data. This underlying infrastructure should be usable in many ways: to identify patients in accordance with their health risk level (high, rising, or low risk), to inform and educate patients, to appropriately organize and deliver medical care, to measure performance, to evaluate the care we are delivering, and to make it as efficient and effective as possible [203].

Data Analytics to Bedside

The BSWQA journey toward population health has involved extensive work to identify patients, engage providers, and measure outcomes in the quest to advance the Triple Aim. Along the way, some of the most innovative work has been centered on population health management specifically related to resource allocation and predictive modeling. BSWQA has increased its investment in Big Data and internally developed predictive analytics to work by refining algorithms to generate actionable predictions.

The genesis of this work is germane to every ACO moving from a fee-for-service to a fee-for-value mission and includes the need to allocate scarce care coordination resources. After having struggled and spent significant hours and intellectual capital investing in vendor- or IT-driven solutions, HTPN partnered with BSWQA to develop an all-disease model of future resource utilization. Guided by the principles of transparency, simplicity, and reproducibility, the team leaned on existing open-source models found in industry-wide literature, in-house subject matter expertise, and award-winning predictive modeling techniques to train and validate its model using objective and subjective approaches.

The models developed leverage nonparametric machine learning algorithms and use patient experiences to train the model. This "more relevant" versus simply "more" training data approach allows the model to reflect the culture, idiosyncrasies, and imperfections of BSWQA patients, providers, and data. These efforts initially targeted high-risk patients—the top 5% attributed to HTPN through its managed care contract agreements including BSWH's employee health plan. Initial success with performing targeted interventions on the top 5% (high-risk) patients was realized. Continued improvement within this high-risk population has allowed progression from a retrospective, reactive model focused on patients who have already had adverse outcomes (top 5%; high risk) to now using predictive modeling where an algorithm is applied to integrated data from multiple sources (inpatient and outpatient EHRs, claims data, and inpatient and outpatient practice management systems) to predict which patients will have adverse outcomes (next 15%; rising risk). The most important factors in the risk model are the number of patients diagnosed with chronic disease, the prior utilization history of a patient, and the number of distinct procedural categories utilized by a patient. Supporting factors include demographic, biometric, socioeconomic, and additional diagnostic and therapeutic signals.

In addition to identifying patients for complex disease management, the predictive model serves to complement existing "hot lists" that identify patients in need of wellness exams and preventive measures. As described earlier in this chapter, patients in the greatest need category—or top 5% (high risk)— are enrolled in complex disease management, medication reconciliation, and transitional care protocols through a nurse care manager. Those identified within the next highest 15% (rising risk) are enrolled in a PCMH approach utilizing transitional care services, and gaps-in-care protocols through a medical assistant health coordinator. Those identified within the lowest (80%) risk are proactively offered wellness and gaps-in-care services. It is in this way that higher quality care is achieved that (1) is wellness oriented and compliant with population contracts, (2) is strategically matched to appropriate care resources to reduce unnecessary, higher-cost interventions, and (3) increases wellness for all populations using a single workflow approach across the risk spectrum (high risk to low risk) (Figure 5.6).

Even with accurate predictions, resource allocation decisions still pose challenges. Of the 750,000 patient encounters

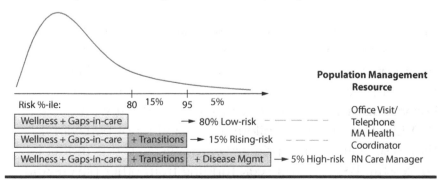

Figure 5.6　Allocating care models in accordance with risk.

within the employed medical group, BSWQA is accountable for the cost and quality of care of more than 300,000 covered lives through participation in particular ACO-based managed care contracts. Assigning care coordination clinical resources to these covered lives becomes a significant computational exercise. Based on an understanding of the importance of the care team to the patient, and optimizing handoffs for clinicians, resources are assigned based on patient-PCP attribution to (1) balance workloads, (2) facilitate enduring relationships, and (3) create geographically contiguous panels to capitalize on research regarding hot spots, food deserts, socioeconomic risks, and so forth.

This success in predictive modeling and resource allocation has not occurred without challenges, past, present, and future. In the design phase, the primary challenges encountered were those of data quality and quantity. In the deployment and scaling phases, the main challenges were tactical in nature, including attribution of patients to providers and assignment of care coordinators to physicians. Ongoing challenges include population and attribution stability and the issue of measuring efficacy over a long term. But fundamentally, this data enable the practitioner and care team to deliver the highest quality, most cost-effective care and to be *accountable* for these outcomes.

Behavioral Health

Mental illnesses such as depression, anxiety, substance abuse, and other serious mental illnesses are a major contributor to health outcomes and cost [27]. In addition, comorbid occurrence of psychological and social issues in association with chronic diseases is common. BSWQA, working with Scott & White Health Plan, is piloting the funding of behavioral therapists within large primary care offices. If this model is successful, BSWQA will seek funding from other payers and employers to help with the management of behavioral health and thereby assist in comprehensively managing all aspects of population health. Behavioral health benefits have often historically been "carved out" in insurance benefit design. It is our strong belief that integrating behavioral care into both primary and specialty care will prove beneficial to patients. BSWQA's close relationship with our provider-ordered plan should help prove this premise.

Value-Based Contracting Driving Improved Quality and Reduced Costs through Population Health Management

BSWQA has experienced early success in accomplishing the Triple Aim as demonstrated by the improved quality and cost outcomes realized from managing the health of the 34,000 enrollees of the BSWH–North Texas division employee health plan. In its first two operational years, BSWQA population health strategies reduced admissions per 1,000, decreased 30-day readmissions, and reduced medical plan costs for the BSWH North Texas division employee health plan by more than 7% for year 1, and 5% for year 2, proving to employers and payers that it has the capacity to generate positive outcomes in an identified patient population. These achievements have prompted the development of BSWQA's compelling story for accountable care driving positive outcomes and true health care transformation through population health management. As the BSWQA accountable care story continues to unfold, payers and employers are taking notice of BSWQA's achievements and seeking collaborative agreements, agreements that are becoming a vital element for creating the value-driven care delivery model of the future. They ask, "Are you really *accountable* for lower cost and improving the health of my employees?" The Baylor Scott & White health care model has been developed and is indicative of the entire clinically integrated program the organization can apply to the patients in any given population.

To effectively manage population health and adapt to the shift in the health care market toward value-based payments and greater provider accountability for quality and cost, BSWQA physicians have the opportunity to participate in shared savings contracts that promote health improvements across populations of patients as well as reductions in health care costs. Contracting with managed care companies in these shared savings agreement opportunities allows BSWQA physicians to utilize risk stratification tools to segment patient populations, reach out to patients who need supplementary care services, and monitor patient populations more efficiently. As of 2015, the BSWQA network was participating in shared savings contract initiatives for more than 300,000 patients of Medicare Advantage and commercial products as well as the MSSP and anticipates growth to more than 500,000 patients by early 2017. BSWH remains in active discussions on behalf of BSWQA with all of the major managed care payers regarding ACO contracting opportunities, such as Medicare Advantage plans and commercial ACO product offerings that will incorporate savings incentives. In addition to incentivizing ACO providers, those savings enable further reinvestment in population health infrastructure and tools. BSWQA further encourages payers and employers to include plan design, incentives for in-network care, wellness incentives, and realistic spending target projections to produce the rewards that both pay for population health program costs and reward providers.

Who Will Benefit from the Baylor Scott & White Health Care Model?

The shared savings bonus percentages reflected in BSWQA's current model emphasizing the role of primary care are not meant to diminish the essential role BSWQA specialists play in

BSWQA's ongoing efforts to improve care delivery and reduce health care costs. In a recent study, BSWQA found that many visits made to specialists after initial referral are for routine or preventive care that could be more cost-effectively delivered through the patient's PCP [204]. Although many ACOs surveyed assign all shared savings to primary care, the BSWQA Finance and Contracting Committee and the board of managers recognized the contribution of both primary care and specialist physicians in the shared savings distribution. Specialists will continue to play an important role in patient care, and ACO primary care participants must have effective working relationships with specialists [205]. For example, whereas some chronic disease patients look to their specialist(s) as their "routine" care providers, opportunities for savings in the primary care model are limited unless specialists are also active participants in holistic care. BSWQA is committed to establishing a balanced environment where primary and specialty care physicians share in savings based on what the BSWQA board of managers believes to be a fair representation of the work that creates that savings, but someone needs to own the comprehensive relationship. While specialty care physicians can impact clinical metrics such as LDL < 100 (cardiologists) or A1C < 7 (endocrinologists), at this time, aligned incentive programs mainly impact quality metrics at the primary care level where the PCP is held *accountable* for reaching quality thresholds as outlined by BSWQA's value-based agreements and employer collaborators. Nevertheless, the BSWQA shared savings bonus distribution model is intended to be fluid and adaptable throughout the years, with distributions changing as specialty metrics evolve and access to more comprehensive and sophisticated data improves. In addition, as the BSWQA becomes more advanced in data analytics (risk stratification and predictive modeling), BSWQA also expects to progress in its ability to measure specific quality, efficiency, and outcome thresholds achieved by both primary and specialty care physicians, and adjudicate rewards in relation to contribution of those who created them.

To be successful in delivering *accountable* care, integrating care into an organized strategy involving health care teams and engaging of BSWQA patients are goals that every primary and specialty physician must endorse. In the first two years of operation with only 34,000 patients, BSWQA specialists have not yet seen significant impact in their patient panels, but the large 2015 growth in contracted lives provides assurance that significant quality referrals to specialists through a more standardized approach to care and improved population health management are rapidly occurring. For example, as PCPs become more fluent in consulting protocols (e.g., the BSWQA low-back-pain protocol), higher-quality appropriate referrals are expected to be directed to their specialty care physician colleagues. Also, PCPs in BSWQA will expect specialists to adhere to the same protocol that they are using.

Optimizing the Medicare Shared Savings Program to Drive Value-Based Care

BSWQA elected initially not to participate in MSSP. Over the past two years, as the organization's population management tools developed, the board of managers felt that the organization was better suited to *successfully* manage MSSP patients. BSWQA was one of 89 ACOs accepted to participate in the MSSP cohort for 2015 [206]. The MSSP is a direct relationship with CMS creating provider member accountability for traditional Medicare beneficiaries as measured by CMS across domains that include specific quality, utilization, and patient experience metrics (see Chapter 3 for more details). BSWQA must achieve a 2% minimum savings rate against the expected spend of the beneficiary population to qualify for shared savings. BSWQA's participation in the MSSP is scheduled to run for three years. Under the MSSP contract, BSWQA is managing the care for 63,000 covered lives.

MSSP ACOs must meet certain quality performance measures with the goal of delivering comprehensive and coordinated patient-centered care [47]. The quality measures emphasize continuous improvement within four domains: patient and caregiver experience, care coordination and patient safety, preventative health, and at-risk populations [49]. Medicare continues to pay fee-for-service payments to individual providers and suppliers for specific items and services. Patients are assigned to MSSP participating providers based on where they receive the majority of their primary care services. If the patient does not have an MSSP PCP, the beneficiary is assigned to a specialist within the ACO where he or she gets the majority of his or her care, but if the patient has seen a PCP in the previous year, efforts are made by care coordination to promote a PCP medical home.

Proactive Customer Engagement: Using a Wellness Visit Business Model to Drive Population Health

Proactive customer engagement using a wellness visit business model for population health is another BSWQA catalyst for further migration from a fee-for-service to fee-for-value workflow. A wellness visit business model increases the network's proficiency in managing the health of patient populations by identifying all the patient's health needs, then utilizing care coordination outreach as a central aspect of proactive customer engagement. Strategic use of care coordinators to schedule office visits generates both fee-for-service revenue and fee-for-value revenue for the provider network and the health system. Each patient within any contracted patient population is scheduled for an annual wellness visit. This is the fundamental approach known as a "wellness visit platform." By establishing a holistic view and comprehensive care plan, coordinated across all disciplines, quality is improved and wasteful cost is averted.

Since the passage of the ACA in 2010, every Medicare beneficiary is eligible for a no-deductible, no-co-pay wellness visit every 12 months in order to facilitate well-being and high-quality health care. The annual wellness visit is an opportunity for appropriate compliance, billing, documentation, and care plan initiation. To create the wellness visit platform, BSWQA utilizes its care coordinators to engage providers with population health education and patients by scheduling proactive appointments. This in turn engages patients in comprehensive care with a primary care provider team. With access to providers' schedules and working off "hot lists" that identify eligible Medicare beneficiaries in need of a wellness visit every 12 months, care coordinators proactively schedule Medicare beneficiaries from the hot lists for their wellness visits. The data analytics team generates hot lists by running risk stratification and predictive modeling algorithms. Medicare beneficiaries eligible for and in need of a wellness visit are ranked "highest risk to lowest risk," with higher-risk patients contacted and scheduled first. To date, care coordinators have scheduled 98% of identified Medicare beneficiaries for their annual wellness visits, with 100% of scheduling expected to be completed by June 30, 2015. By proactively scheduling patients for their wellness visits, illness burdens can be accurately documented, quality metrics can be completed, and gaps in care can be closed before critical events occur. Care then improves and wasteful costs are avoided.

By the end of 2014, through the strategic use of care coordinators, BSWQA attained an impressive increase in the number of annual wellness visits, resulting in an initial increase in revenue to PCPs from $30,000 to more than $300,000 through the following mechanisms:

■ Provider engagement and education regarding annual wellness visits
■ Proactive scheduling of annual wellness visits by care coordinators
■ Clinical workflow efficiencies during the visit itself

- Revenue capture for annual wellness visits
- Clinical documentation improvement using annual wellness visits and standardized EHR templates
- Growing provider understanding of wellness assessment as a basis for chronic disease management
- More accurate, complete coding and risk adjustment factor (RAF) score optimization

How the Wellness Visit Business Model Works

A wellness visit business model using proactive patient engagement encourages patient-centeredness. It engages providers to manage a population of patients in a manner that increases quality, decreases unnecessary overall cost, and increases patient satisfaction. Within the Medicare beneficiary annual wellness visit, the provider is able to deliver and document all 33 quality metrics associated with both traditional MSSP and Medicare Advantage value-based contract requirements. In addition, the annual wellness visit provides a vehicle for documenting the hierarchical condition category (HCC) codes necessary to establish the risk status (RAF score) of the patient to the highest degree of specificity. HCCs are an important component for determining the true risk status of the patient so that funds can be appropriately received for the level of care necessary to manage the patient. Honing these skills within Medicare contracts has prepared providers for proficiently managing the health of patient populations as well as those assigned by current and future Medicare Advantage and commercial contracts. To help its providers refine these skills, BSWQA's performance management team defined five clinical factors for population health management success that can be driven by the wellness visit business model:

1. **Transparency (data):** The annual wellness visit is a vehicle for complete and accurate documentation of all medical conditions in a proper manner that can be reported and shared.

2. **Engagement:** Data captured during the annual wellness visit allow for accurate predictive analysis on future health services needed so care coordination and any needed resources can be employed.

3. **Stabilization:** The annual wellness visit sets the scenario for routine care with a PCP team, stabilizing the patient within the network. This in essence stabilizes the network's patient base within the contracts and grows market share.

4. **Optimization:** The annual wellness visit offers a systematic means for documenting discrete data that optimizes opportunities for taking care of the "whole" patient.

5. **Variation reduction:** Annual wellness visits systemize a "best practice" approach for documentation that is leveraged throughout the system, reducing variability.

Process Design

The multidisciplinary team heading this project utilized the Accelerating Best Care (ABC) improvement process developed by BSWH and is based on both rapid-cycle improvement and Lean methodology. It is designed to rapidly spread quality improvement initiatives throughout the organization. The team implemented the plan, do, check, act cycle of change of the rapid-cycle method and measured the impact of the newly designed or redesigned process over a short period of time.

■ **Plan:** The scope of this project reflects the organization's focus on comprehensive care management with access and appropriate documentation of diagnosis codes within a patient's record and claims. The issues were identified using the brainstorming model. Together, the flow diagram (Figure 5.7) and interrelationship digraph (Figure 5.8) suggested that the team focus on provider and staff training and core processes of practice workflow, resulting in ideal documentation.

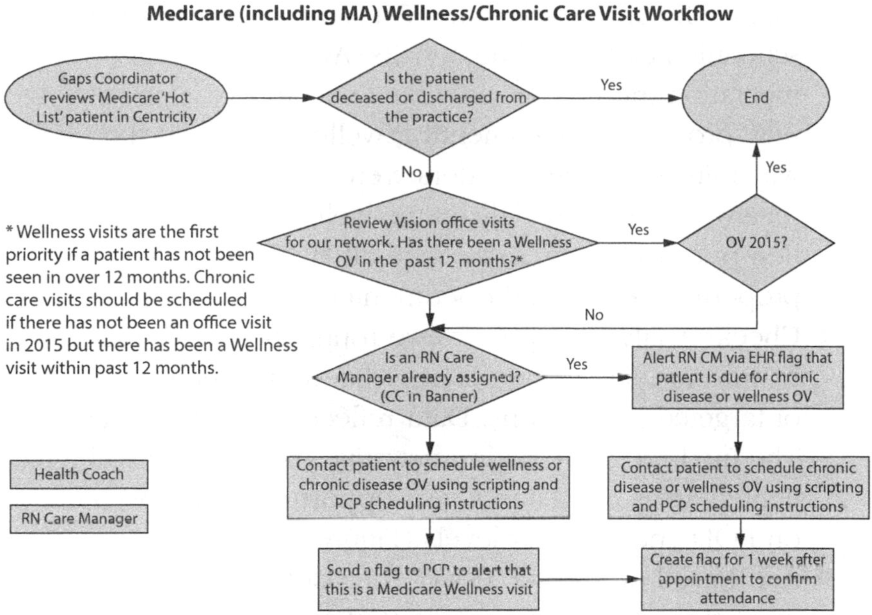

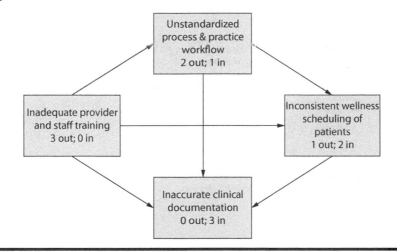

Medicare (including MA) Wellness/Chronic Care Visit Workflow

Figure 5.7   Medicare wellness visit workflow.

Figure 5.8   Interrelationship diagraph.

■ **Do:** The proposed plan was implemented in phases, starting with care coordinators receiving access to physician schedules in order to schedule wellness visits for a pilot group of provider champions. Physicians historically are reluctant to give others access to their schedules, but today 62% of physicians in HTPN allow schedulers to schedule needed wellness visits. An emphasis on documentation training for providers was the next priority. A new process for documenting wellness visits in the EHR was initiated. Finally, coders were hired and trained to review all Medicare Advantage wellness visits documentation prior to billing, to be sure all HCC conditions were properly assessed and documented.

■ **Check:** Analytics reports were routinely pulled from the EHR to measure progress on scheduling wellness visits of targeted populations. Data reflect favorable results. The medical group's administrative dashboard also highlighted areas of wellness visit opportunity improvement on POD and provider levels (Figure 5.9).

■ **Act:** Based on the success of the pilot intervention, process improvements were adopted and spread across the network's patient populations and practices.

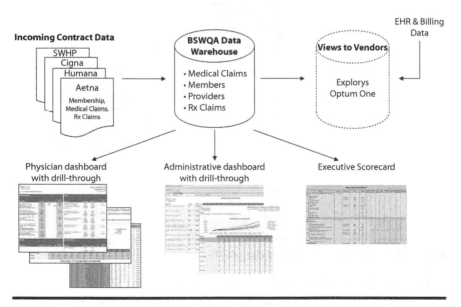

Figure 5.9 Administrative dashboard data architecture. Note: SWHP = Scott & White Health Plan; BSWQA = Baylor Scott & White Quality Alliance; EHR = electronic health record.

Deployment

Deployment of the wellness visit platform began with enterprise-wide provider engagement that included gaining permission for care coordinators to have access to providers' schedules so that wellness scheduling could be initiated. After an eight-week pilot period was implemented with select physician champions from the organization's Disease Management Committee, lunchtime site visits to each of the adult primary care ambulatory sites (more than 50 different sites) began. "Hot lists" identifying eligible Medicare beneficiaries in need of a wellness visit within 12 months were generated from Medicare Advantage contracts, and chronic disease visits were generated for commercial contracts.

In addition to the lunchtime site visits, providers were offered and strongly encouraged to attend wellness visit educational training sessions. These sessions were held within each geographic POD region as well as posted online to give providers a virtual training option. Providers who attended the training were given continuing medical education (CME) credit, and in January 2015 these training sessions became a requirement for clinical integration as outlined by the BSWQA shared savings distribution model. More than 300 providers attended these training sessions in person.

A practice management system software deficiency was discovered that limited an office visit billing to only four diagnosis codes, and a work-around was identified to submit up to the allowed 12 codes per visit when appropriate. This became known as the additional code diagnosis process. More than 70,000 office visits in 2014 for traditional Medicare were affected and supplemental codes submitted.

The annual wellness visit is also an effective vehicle for improving clinical documentation, which includes complete and proper coding and diagnosis reporting. Complete clinical documentation tells the patient's entire health story and is used to ensure that his or her disease burden is accurately reported so that reimbursements as well as the care resources are allocated appropriately. The impact of complete or incomplete documentation behavior skews the risk stratification and predictive modeling used to allocate care resources. Without documenting the condition codes correctly, the risk stratification tool is not as accurate as it could be, and therefore care management is not as efficient.

Clinical documentation, specifically the nuances of HCC coding, is time-consuming as well as challenging to learn and understand for clinical provide teams. A clinical documentation improvement program was initiated with enterprise-wide education while HCC coding documentation experts began to retrospectively review 2014 records. Developing system-level workflows that scale required the initiation of training for provider clinical teams, operational teams, and revenue cycle management teams, including charge entry staff, beginning in October 2014.

Using a Wellness Visit Business Model to Transform Health Care

Wellness visit business models proactively facilitate patient engagement with clinical teams, streamline the patient clinical experience, establish patient personalized health goals related to known chronic conditions (diabetes, blood pressure, heart failure, emphysema, and asthma), and create a well-being preventive plan of care. Wellness visit business models also simultaneously facilitate the clinical team's ability to identify patient barriers to wellness, including patients' management of their health, patients' access to care, family support deficiencies, and lack of community resources.

The current model of health care delivery is unsustainable and at times is broken. MSSP and other value-based population health contracts are just the beginning steps to improving care delivery. Those who *provide the care* have the chance to advocate for *those who need the care* in a manner that truly provides the right care in the right way at the right time for the right patient. Participating in contracts like MSSP and applying a wellness model to the populations that are served gives BSWQA the opportunity to truly transform health care.

Information Technology: Promoting Population Health

Electronic Health Record

The EHR is a critical component of BSWQA's drive toward clinical integration. It allows BSWQA physicians to better coordinate and manage the care of their patients, and also serves as the gateway for patient information sharing. The BSWQA IT (Informatics) Committee is charged with administering processes for patient information sharing by optimizing EHR utilization throughout the BSWQA provider community so that relevant data can be accurately extracted from various data sources including physician offices, hospitals, and outpatient facilities. The Committee has made significant progress in advancing toward a "connected network of providers." To ensure complete sharing of patient information, BSWQA requires all physician members to implement and utilize a Certification Commission for Healthcare Information Technology (CCHIT) approved EHR that qualifies users for meaningful use, but also incorporates certain connectivity and interoperability standards.

Data acquired in the EHR are aggregated within the HIE primarily out of continuity of care document (CCD) or clinical document architecture (CDA), which is standardized nationally but can still vary slightly across EHRs dependent on how the physician is entering information. The CCD or CDA provides visibility into how the physician is utilizing the EHR. For example, physicians have a responsibility to maintain adequate problem lists, perform medication reconciliation, and review and update allergy lists. If physicians are not appropriately maintaining these things, it limits the ability to collect comparative data. In addition, BSWQA physicians must be able to recognize who their ACO patients are. To assist with recognizing BSWQA patients, a BSWQA *patient identifier* has been put into the headers of the various EHRs in use throughout the BSWQA network. With the BSWQA patient identifier, physicians will be able to readily identify a patient as a BSWQA member who therefore has access to enhanced care management services through the BSWQA care coordination department. For example, if a BSWQA patient goes to the ED, a physician may be more willing to send that patient home knowing that a BSWQA care coordinator will be available to assist in the transition from hospital to home through follow-up phone calls and assurance that an appointment will be scheduled for that patient. Without being identified, and absent the consequent assurance of timely follow-up, the physician may feel compelled to admit that patient to the hospital or order a 24-hour observation that is costly to both the patient and the system.

Future plans include making the patient's "risk category" visible in the BSWQA identifier. For instance, a high-risk (top 5%) patient will be identified as BSWQA5, a rising-risk (15%) patient will be identified as BSWQA15, and a low-risk (80%) patient will identified as BSWQA80. With this additional knowledge at their fingertips, physicians can better allocate care resources appropriately for that patient.

Health Information Exchange

One of BSWQA's biggest challenges as an organization is connectivity. Although the 1,800 employed BSWH physicians will be on a single EHR, to date there are 76 different EHRs being utilized throughout the BSWQA network by over 2,200 independent physicians. To achieve a fully connected network,

BSWQA began an evaluation and selection process on a number of HIE vendors. HIE vendor selection criteria revolved around (1) flexibility in attaining connectivity among a large variety of EHRs and (2) the vendor's ability to attain connectivity quickly because of the rapidly growing ACO patient population.

Upon completion of a number of vendor evaluations, dbMotion™ was selected based on its high KLAS ranking as well as its demonstrated ability to implement connectivity quickly (Figure 5.10) [207].

KLAS is an independently owned and operated company that aims to improve health care technology by measuring vendor performance for its provider partners [208]. The vendor selection was approved by the BSWQA board of managers as well as BSWH system leadership and the board of trustees. Once approval from both boards was finalized, a plan was launched by the BSWQA IT Committee to begin connectivity among all of BSWH facilities and all of the ambulatory clinics, which would result in achieving approximately 80% connectivity across BSWQA. Complete connectivity is on track to be performed over a two-year period and completed by early 2016, which in the IT industry is considered to be a rapid pace for connectivity and implementation.

dbMotion facilitates interoperability and HIE for health information networks and integrated health care delivery systems. The service-oriented architecture (SOA)–based dbMotion solution gives caregivers and information systems secure access to an integrated patient record composed from a patient's medical data maintained at facilities that are otherwise unconnected or have no common technology through which to share data, without requiring the replacement of existing information systems. dbMotion can interoperate with multiple different vendor products, and the architecture's modularity allows for multiple approaches to sharing medical information (i.e., centralized, distributed or federated, or any hybrid format). It can aggregate the clinical vocabulary, or semantics, from disparate systems from different vendors,

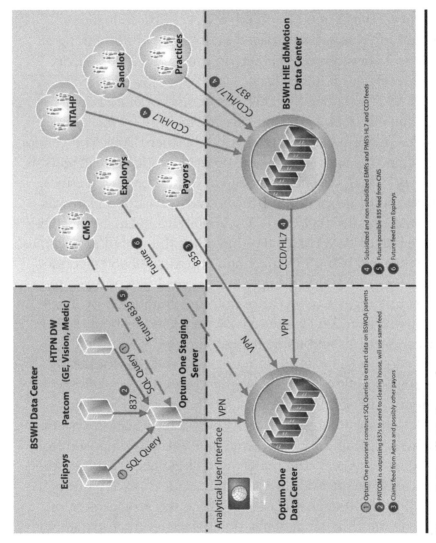

Figure 5.10   dbMotion schema.

making it possible to view all medication orders across intensive care unit (ICU), ED, medical and surgical units, and ambulatory environments, and integrate them into a simplified clinical summary. The use of interoperability can enhance efficiency and improve quality of care.

In accountable care, data are needed for two purposes: care and performance. dbMotion is a critical element of the connectivity plan within BSWQA. In addition to connecting the differing EHRs, it will also furnish data to BSWQA data analytic systems. An important key feature of dbMotion is a delta agent, which resides within the EHR. This agent captures existing patient information that does not currently reside in the physician's EHR and presents it in a concise and useful manner. For instance, if a patient was seen in an urgent care center or had specific diagnostics, labs, or x-rays done, the HIE delta agent will deliver that information to the physician's EHR in the form of a pop-up window. The physician will be prompted and asked whether he or she would like to accept the information and add it to the patient's EHR. This agent does not require going out to a separate website, making it extremely simple to use. The delta agent helps to provide an all-inclusive view of the patient, keeping the physician better informed and able to make appropriate decisions, devise more accurate treatment plans, and avoid duplicate or redundant testing. The all-inclusive view also enables physicians to be *accountable* to the information they may not have had at their fingertips in the past. In knowing a patient's full health history, a physician can begin to see the segments of the patient population that represent gaps in care or recognize a patient who may be at very high risk and has not had a physician visit. As the patient's data is aggregated by the HIE and reviewed by staff, the patient can be proactively contacted utilizing various BSWQA population health resources to connect the patient with a PCP and address some of the barriers the patient may have to accessing care.

As the HIE is deployed, the prioritization is on practices and facilities that have a large number of BSWQA patients while simultaneously attempting to align with BSWQA population health strategies. By collecting patient information and building the capability for patient information sharing among all BSWQA providers, dbMotion offers an exciting opportunity to collect rich data in the form of a patient's medical history, risk status, cost, and more. Providing physicians with a more comprehensive view of patient information gives them the tools they need to take a more *accountable*, proactive, comprehensive approach to care, both from a clinical standpoint and with consideration of cost.

Population Health: Summary

Accountability and improving population health are centered not only on how well an ACO can build the right infrastructure, but also on changes in how care is delivered at the practitioner level. To be successful, both the organization and its individual members must be *accountable*. In transforming health care, we are attempting to move from a fee-for-service, reactive model of care where we see patients only when they are ill to a care model that utilizes population health resources such as PCMHs, disease management, preventive care, and evidence-based protocols, care coordination, data analytics, and health informatics to move the entire patient population toward better health. One major goal is to establish the PCP as the care management anchor to maintain the health of patients and manage them in a way that they are able to reduce their disease burdens. Proactively reaching out to patients enables health systems to perform routine care, keeps the patients in line of sight, fills the care gaps where necessary, educates the patients and teaches them to navigate the system, and potentially deploys appropriate care interventions before the patient has an event. Empowering patients to understand what they need, when they need it, and why they need it improves not only the quality of care, but also, more importantly, their quality of life. Care coordinators, data analytics, PCMHs, wellness programs, and even reward systems are not enough to achieve better population health. In addition to the infrastructure described in this section, physician engagement and *accountability* is essential.

Chapter 6

Financing Accountable Care

Main Points for Chapter

This chapter includes a discussion of:

- Health care cost sustainability and drivers of rising health care costs
- Ways to improve health care value by reducing waste
- How accountable care organizations enable participants to share in rewards for improved quality and efficiency while reducing costs
- Alternative payment models such as value-based purchasing and bundled payments
- The role of employers in funding health insurance redesign

Health Care Costs

Because health care costs are too high, reducing per capita health care costs is one of the three goals of the Triple Aim.

ACOs have the potential to lower costs, but financing accountable care is challenging in a health care system that has typically focused on treatment rather than prevention and has
been shaped by the fee-for-service payment model. Factors
like evolving technology, poor coordination between unconnected care sites, poor end-of-life care, and an aging population more susceptible to chronic diseases have further driven
costs to unsustainable levels (Chapter 2).

Researchers and critics of the U.S. health care system have
noted that differences in health care costs often fail to reflect
differences in health care quality [209]. For example, regional
variation in health care spending has been found to be associated with neither quality of care nor access to care—although
some of these differences can be explained by other factors,
such as more inpatient-based and specialist-oriented patterns
of practice in high-spending areas [210, 211]. In addition,
health care prices are usually not transparent to consumers
because insurance plans, benefit structures, and health
care plan features such as deductibles and co-pays obscure
cost differences (see Chapter 4). Variation in health care
costs coupled with a lack of price transparency have led to
uncertainty among consumers and payers about the actual
value of some health care services.

The current state of economics in the United States and the
difficulty in achieving population health have further been
compounded by the traditional fee-for-service payment model.
The "more is better" provider and physician payments do not
necessarily lead to better long-term health outcomes, and in
fact the opposite is true: states with the highest CMS spending
per beneficiary have the poorest health outcomes. "More" is
not better care (Figure 2.5) [38]. Fee-for-service payment mechanisms often fail to reimburse providers for the time and coor-
dinative resources required to manage the health of patients
with multiple or complex conditions. For example, a physician
may not be able to afford to take the time to help patients
understand why a certain expensive procedure or test is not

needed [212]. In some cases, it is easier and more time efficient to simply order the test. Compounding that fact, the physician may be paid *more* for ordering the unneeded test. Because of the crucial role of physician decision making in determining and recommending appropriate procedures, tests, and interventions for patients, transforming the U.S. health care system into an ***accountable*** one that rewards value will require strong physician leadership as well as a more widespread understanding of the role of factors that influence physician judgment and treatment recommendations [213, 214]. Changing the way health care is delivered and reimbursed to emphasize value over volume is challenging but essential to improving accountable care.

In addition to health care payment mechanisms, the aging of the U.S. population is another important driver of rising costs. The cost of providing health care for one person age 65 or older has been estimated to be three to five times higher than the cost for someone younger than 65, and the CDC has suggested that by 2030, without taking into account inflation and the higher costs of new technology, health care spending will increase by 25%, just because the population will be older [215]. A result of the aging U.S. population is the high cost of care for patients at the end of life. About one-quarter of Medicare's annual budget has been estimated to fund care for patients during their final year of life [216], although end-of-life treatment is often intensive, futile, and unwanted by many patients who prefer hospice or home care [11]. Simple advanced planning can avert much of that futile care, yet advanced planning by practitioners spending needed time with patients is both time-consuming and poorly reimbursed in a fee-for-service world.

Redundancy, care fragmentation, and poor flow of data between care sites are additional contributors to rising health care costs; enhancing care coordination through technology is essential to improving accountability for and quality of health care [6, 58]. As discussed in Chapter 4, ACOs encourage stronger alignment of quality goals and metrics across inpatient and outpatient settings by allocating the savings that are shared when quality health care is delivered at lower costs by requiring their participants to achieve or exceed specific quality metrics and by integrating goals, initiatives, and metrics between hospital care and ambulatory care settings. This integration depends in part on the development and implementation of HIT infrastructure and HIE, which have enormous potential to enhance coordination of care across different providers and sites. Payers and policy makers have recognized this potential, and currently, the meaningful use of EHRs is a prerequisite for eligible professionals and hospitals to qualify for CMS incentive programs. In this context, "meaningful use" is defined as the use of certified EHR technology to improve quality, safety, and efficiency, and reduce health disparities; engage patients and families; improve care coordination and population and public health; and maintain privacy and security of patient health information [217].

Widespread HIT adoption is facilitating improvements in health services delivery as well as spurring innovations in payment methods, and has been found specifically to improve delivery of care based on guidelines (particularly in preventive health), enhance monitoring and surveillance activities, reduce medication errors, and decrease rates of utilization for potentially redundant or inappropriate care [218]. However, adoption of HIT such as EHR systems can lead to higher short-term costs related to acquisition, staffing, productivity, and training [219, 220]. EHRs have a major influence on physician satisfaction as well, and many physicians have felt that EHRs negatively impact their workflows. Thus, rapidly changing technology is an important driver of rising health care costs—even as EHRs and related technology are expected to mitigate these costs in the long term.

Improving Health Care Value by Reducing Waste

Summarizing the opportunity to bring health care costs into a sustainable range for patients and payers, Berwick and Hackbarth described the following six forms of wasteful (i.e., non-value-added) care and estimated that the sum of the lowest available estimates for these six forms of waste exceeds 20% of total health care expenditures [11]:

- **Failures of care delivery:** The waste that comes with poor execution or lack of widespread adoption of known best-care processes, including, for example, patient safety systems and preventive care practices that have been shown to be effective.
- **Failures of care coordination:** The waste that comes when patients fall through the gaps in fragmented care. The results are complications, hospital readmissions, declines in functional status, and increased dependency, especially for the chronically ill.
- **Overtreatment:** The waste that comes from subjecting patients to care that, according to sound science and the patients' own preferences, cannot possibly help them. Examples include excessive use of antibiotics, use of surgery when watchful waiting is better, and unwanted intensive care at the end of life for patients who prefer hospice and home care.
- **Administrative complexity:** The waste that comes when government, accreditation agencies, payers, and others create inefficient or misguided rules. For example, payers may fail to standardize forms, thereby consuming limited physician time in needlessly complex billing procedures.
- **Pricing failures:** The waste that comes as prices migrate far from those expected in well-functioning markets, that is, the actual costs of production plus a fair profit. For example, because of the absence of effective transparency and competitive markets, U.S. prices for diagnostic procedures such as MRI and computed tomography (CT) scans are several times more than those of identical procedures in other countries.

■ **Fraud and abuse:** The waste that comes as fraudsters issue fake bills and run scams, and also from the blunt procedures of inspection and regulation that everyone faces because of the misbehaviors of a very few.

Currently, the Dallas–Fort Worth area is one of the higher health care cost areas in the nation, with overall clinical outcomes no better than seen in areas that deliver care at lower cost [221]. Physicians in high-spending regions see patients return more frequently and are more likely to recommend screening tests of unproven benefit and perform discretionary interventions than physicians in low-spending regions; however, both appear equally likely to recommend guideline-supported interventions [214]. This information suggests that the opportunity exists in the broader market within which BSWQA physicians serve for physicians and hospitals to produce better value (i.e., achieve better health outcomes per dollar spent, measured over the patient's entire care cycle) [19, 40, 121].

Physicians are generally enthusiastic about the ideas of improving value by reducing or eliminating waste, but seldom see themselves as individually wasting health care dollars. Frequently, waste is seen as both nebulous and stemming from the bureaucratic and regulatory burdens that have become endemic in medicine—in other words, not areas likely to be affected by individual action. The six forms of waste identified by Berwick and Hackbarth, however, all include aspects that fall within the control of both individual clinicians and health care provider organizations [11]. For an individual physician to acknowledge that he or she is actually a part of excessive cost, and to be *accountable* for lowering that cost, is disruptive and goes against raw self-interest.

While ACOs are unlikely to have much impact on the time and money spent on preventing and detecting fraud and abuse, they do have the potential to impact the other five forms of waste: ACOs that negotiate on behalf of networks of providers that hold meaningful proportions of the local market share will have bargaining power to influence such things as the administrative procedures of contracting payers and pricing of ancillary services. Even more significantly, however, they can address the failures of care delivery and coordination and overtreatment through their internal mechanisms—including performance measurement, shared savings, and care coordination. While the providers within the ACO might think of the actions taken in these areas as improving the quality of the care they provide, a benefit of that improvement is reduced waste. For example, consider the following example of Mrs. A's experience of care and the associated costs under the current fragmented health care system versus within an ACO that has established the same type of infrastructure as BSWQA:

> Mrs. A was admitted to the emergency room after she fainted. Her blood pressure on admission was 70/30 mmHg and her blood potassium level was 2.0 mg/dL but when she regained consciousness she reported having a history of hypertension. Hearing this, Dr. C, her emergency department physician, suspected an overdose of her antihypertensive medication as the most likely cause of her current hypotension and low potassium. After questioning her further, he learned that she was unable to access her PCP so she had recently visited a cardiologist for her hypertension and that he had changed her medication to a brand-named combination of reserpine and a diuretic. As recommended, Mrs. A had been prescribed an initial reserpine dose of 0.5 mg orally once a day for the first week, but her prescription had not been lowered to the 0.1 mg once a day maintenance dose thereafter. She had started feeling dizzy a few days previously and had started cutting her dose in half, but had not contacted either her cardiologist or pharmacist. The cumulative overdose she had taken over this time resulted in the costly emergency room

visit—and forced her to cancel the movers she had scheduled to be at her house that day.

Consider what Mrs. A's experience should look like in an ACO like BSWQA that has established the infrastructure to coordinate care and encourage disease management for patients with chronic conditions like hypertension. In BSWQA, Mrs. A would have had access to a PCP in a PCMH—and as part of that physician acquiring and maintaining his or her PCMH accreditation (a coming condition for membership in BSWQA), the primary care practice would maintain levels of access and communication that should encourage Mrs. A to seek hypertension care there, rather than seeing a cardiologist for routine hypertension management. On the physician's side of this coin, the BSWQA shared savings program also encourages Mrs. A's PCP to manage her hypertension within the primary care setting where he or she can comprehensively influence the other aspects of Mrs. A's care that are reflected in the shared savings performance measures, as well as the cost of her care (including the immediate reduction in cost by avoiding the more expensive specialist time). Further, the standard BSWQA protocol for hypertension management would not have included reserpine as a first-line pharmaceutical choice, and should even be avoided in the elderly.

Other differences that the BSWQA model facilitates include greater likelihood, with the after-hours access and options of prompt telephonic and electronic communication required by the PCMH standards, that Mrs. A would contact her PCP or care team in the event that a new medication caused persistent dizziness rather than attempting to deal with the problem herself by halving the dose. Finally, it is likely in a PCMH that patients who are being prescribed a new medication would be flagged in the EHR for follow-up by members of the care coordination team to ensure both that the patient had correctly understood the dosing instructions and that she was not experiencing any serious adverse effects. In the case of medication regimens that included a switch from an initial or loading dose to a maintenance dose without another office visit, this protocol would likely include scheduling a second follow-up at the time of that switch to ensure it was made correctly.

All these differences are about improving the quality of care Mrs. A receives, but in addition to the health benefit she receives from the better-coordinated care, it is clear that substantial costs are being avoided: not only does Mrs. A avoid a costly ED visit and cancellation of her movers, but the costs of her dual office visits for hypertension can be decreased by managing her condition in a primary rather than specialty care setting. Further, her medication costs may be reduced if the cardiologist does not prescribe a brand-name drug when the BSWQA standards call for use of a generic.

In the discussion of waste, however, a fact that cannot be avoided is that one person's waste is someone else's income and profit. In the scenario above, the savings in Mrs. A's care are, under a fee-for-service reimbursement mechanism, losses in revenue to Dr. C, the hospital, and the manufacturer of any brand name medication. Shared savings are intended to mitigate those losses for Dr. C and the hospital, but they are unlikely to equal the profits they would have made, as the savings are offset by compensation to the PCP and the care coordinators for the time spent on the nonbillable care for Mrs. A that enabled those savings. The better form of mitigation ACOs can offer specialists and hospitals is "replacement volume": as the "per person" demand for specialist and inpatient care decreases under the influence of the ACO's care coordination and population health activities, more "persons" are needed to keep the specialists and hospitals operating at a financially viable capacity. ACOs provide these persons by expanding their contracted population and by creating systems that encourage referral to the in-network specialists and hospitals when care in those settings is genuinely needed. Even such replacement volume has its limits, though, dictated by the size of the population in the area served and the market share the ACO controls. Nonetheless, high value has attracted market share in all sectors of the economy, including health care.

Ultimately, this model likely may result in a fundamental shift in the U.S. health care system, with more physicians training in and practicing primary care versus entering the currently more prestigious and profitable specialties, and reductions in the numbers of hospitals and staffed beds within hospitals. It would be naïve to think that such changes can be achieved without some stakeholders who enjoyed comfortable profits under the fee-for-service system experiencing losses, but the alternative is to allow current momentum to carry the U.S. health care system into a tragedy of the commons in which individual stakeholders, acting independently and rationally according to their own self-interest, behave contrary to the best interests of the whole group by depleting a common resource [222]. The challenge, therefore, is to ensure that changes happen in such a way as to ensure that what is retained is the high-quality provision of necessary and beneficial care, while what is reduced is poor quality, unnecessary, or inappropriate services (i.e., waste). This requires that diverse and, in some cases, historically adversarial stakeholders like payers and providers work together to coordinate concomitant shifts in the care model and reimbursement mechanism from volume based to value based. Some of these stakeholders may have to act against their own short-term interests to preserve the overall long-term benefits. This movement is complicated even further by the involvement of corporate and publicly traded stakeholders, whose duties to their shareholders may limit their abilities to take such actions.

Current and Future Role of Payers

The growth of accountable care is creating a transformation in the way health care is financed, including the adoption of reimbursement models that emphasize value over volume.

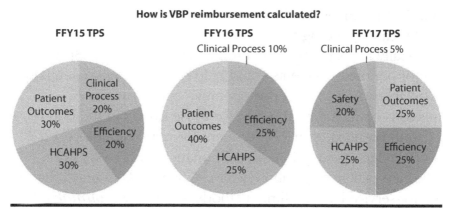

How is VBP reimbursement calculated?

Figure 6.1   Value-based purchasing.

The CMS Hospital Value-Based Purchasing (VBP) Program offers one example of this shift to a stronger focus on quality of care [185]. To facilitate the delivery of value-based care, CMS provides financial incentives to hospitals based on how closely they follow best clinical practices, enhance the patient experience of care, improve health outcomes and patient safety, and rely on efficient practices. Figure 6.1 provides a more detailed description of how VBP reimbursement is calculated. Hospitals receive a total performance score based on specific measures of care quality, such as reductions in health care–acquired infections, delivery of clinical processes associated with better health care outcomes, and performance across measures of patient experience. A certain percentage of hospital reimbursement is then linked to this score. The tying of the total performance score to financial payment fosters hospital and provider accountability for the health, outcomes, and overall experience of patients.

A "bundled payment" approach is another example of a payment mechanism that rewards value and quality over volume of services provided and encourages *accountability* for outcomes. A bundled payment provides a single payment by the payer for all services related to a given treatment or condition, thereby encouraging both hospital and physician providers to assume part of the risk for preventable health care costs.

Bundled payments could provide a mechanism for reducing health care spending through improved care coordination, especially for patients with chronic conditions [38, 223]. The use of bundled payments could help to discourage potentially avoidable costs, such as postoperative complications or read-missions by including the care for those events in the bundle.

In the context of ACOs, payment for value is often based on providers' assumption of some financial risk for account-able care patient population health. While an ACO may rely on fee-for-service-based billing methods, it is also *accountable* for maintaining and enhancing the health of attributed patients over time. Types of ACO payment arrangements can include (1) capi-tation (global payments for the health care needs of the ACO patient population), (2) bundled payments, (3) shared savings (using fee-for-service payments as a basis, but with retrospective reward or penalties if the total annual cost for a population is more or less than certain targets), and (4) pay-for-performance models, which allow providers to receive bonus payments or increases in their base fee schedule that are conditioned on reaching performance benchmarks [50]. The first three payment arrangements listed entail some provider assumption of finan-cial risk for ACO patient population health [53]. The BSWQA also operates under the MSSP model (described in more detail in Chapters 4 and 5). However, successful ACOs will by neces-sity begin to accept financial risk for the cost of care as well as the quality. BSWQA is committed to that transition over time.

Financing Population Health

Defining the Patient Population

ACOs need to ensure their providers have the tools to be *accountable* and that they understand for what and for whom they are accountable. For example, as members in good standing with BSWQA, providers have voluntarily agreed in their signed participation agreements to be accountable for clinical integration, quality, efficiency (reducing cost), and the patient experience—all in terms of providing care for a population of patients. In the ACO world, that population is most likely attributed to the organization through managed care commercial contracts, Medicare Advantage contracts, or the MSSP. ACOs are financially accountable for all the care delivered to their attributed patients, whether the care is delivered by ACO members, contracted providers, or noncontracted providers [50].

Traditionally, providers deliver care to one patient during one office visit at a time. In population health delivery, in contrast, providers are accountable for delivering quality, efficient care to an attributed population that includes patients they already see (or have seen) and those they have not seen. Proactively engaging those patients thought to be at risk, scheduling them to be seen by physicians, and bringing them into care management are critical. Health risk assessments and biometric screenings performed as a separate event or as part of a wellness visit at the onset of managing any contracted population help providers to identify those with manageable risks. Additionally, especially in chronic disease management, the off-radar management of patients by nurses and others can be as important as physician visits [81].

Patient populations in the commercial space are sometimes acquired through insurance products that utilize very specific provider networks commonly known as "narrow networks." These narrow network arrangements contain benefit designs such as lower co-pays, which incentivize "in-network" utilization. For example, the plan might pay 90% after a deductible to those who utilize providers in network and might pay a much lower percentage for those who seek care from a provider who is "out of network." Patient populations in the commercial space are considered "assigned" to providers by the health plan dependent on whether or not the physician is a participating provider in the narrow network.

These types of value-based preferred-network contracts are gaining popularity among payers and employers as they are viewed as a way to control cost and ensure quality over time [224].

Sharing in Rewards for Improved Quality and Efficiency While Reducing Costs

Members of BSWQA have agreed to share *accountability* for efficiency and quality performance across the network. As a result of these efforts, BSWQA members are eligible to share cost savings realized by contracted payers. In its efforts toward clinical integration, BSWQA is prepared to measure and monitor network success in (1) enhancing clinical outcomes, (2) improving patient safety, (3) adopting clinical technology, (4) improving patient satisfaction, and (5) increasing efficiency. BSWQA's accomplishment of these aims has resulted in cost efficiencies, and therefore the potential for savings to share.

After review by a multispecialty physician finance and contracting committee and the BSWQA board of managers, a working model was approved for the distribution of potential shared savings bonuses (Chapter 4). This model is reviewed annually as BSWQA acquires more sophisticated clinical data to better measure quality and efficiencies. Pending the acquisition of such data, the committee chose to utilize a combination of panel size based on BSWQA attribution as well as pro rata basis within the respective primary care and specialty care pools for the final tier of the distribution method. However, the "panel size" metric encourages PCPs to actively manage and meet the needs of patients in their panels. In BSWQA, "covered lives" is growing in importance to both our physicians and hospitals.

The "Why" Behind the BSWQA Shared Savings Bonus Distribution

The "why" behind BSWQA's shared savings bonus percentages lies in today's health care delivery focus that is rapidly shifting responsibility to the PCPs, widely considered to be the first stop for lowering health care costs as they manage complex disease, wellness, and prevention. These comprehesive efforts sometimes translate into unbillable and uncompensated work at the primary care level, work that is historically outside of the PCP's traditional scope of practice. All of these new expectations occur in the face of an ongoing PCP shortage throughout the United States [225]. Research shows that shared savings should be allocated based on the level of physician ability to affect cost control, care quality, and care coordination. In BSWQA, the organization has determined that the PCP has the most effective opportunity to control these tasks and therefore should receive a higher percentage of any shared savings bonus [226].

In addition, distributing a higher shared savings bonus percentage to PCPs advances BSWQA's commitment to building a solid network of PCMHs, and this is considered to be a key strategy for achieving true clinical integration [227]. With BSWQA specialty physician membership currently outnumbering PCPs, it is BSWQA's hope that creating an opportunity for PCPs to attain increased compensation will incent them to join or become BSWQA PMCHs, and this will result in boosting PCP membership, increasing opportunity for appropriate referrals to BSWQA specialists and contributing to the overall growth of BSWQA.

BSWH is aggressively intending to boost primary care capacity by creating incentives for PCPs to expand their teams with nurse practitioners and physician assistants, expanding programs for PCP residency training, and better rewarding PCPs who can take the expanded responsibilities of being a team manager and "comprehensivist."

Payers and providers are well aware that a strong accountable PCP base will enable superior cost and quality care delivery. BSWQA's continued efforts to develop a strong foundation of BSWQA PCPs will therefore aid in attracting prominent commercial payers and regional employers to contract in aligned incentive programs such as value-based agreements. Aligned incentive programs and value-based agreements help BSWQA to attract patient populations, as illustrated by the rapid growth in covered lives.

Employer-Financed Insurance and Insurance Design

Employers fund much of the commercial health insurance in the United States. Many large employers' health insurance plans are self-funded; others buy fully funded coverage from connected carriers. Given the large proportion of time most adults spend in the workplace, employers have an important role to play in disease prevention through ensuring that workplaces are safe and enable employee access to key determinants of health, such as affordable healthy food choices at the workplace and locations where they can be physically active. Employers can also offer wellness programs and health insurance incentives that encourage employees to incorporate healthy living into their workday and lifestyle [228]. The BSWQA annual wellness visit program described in Chapter 5 offers one example of a model for such initiatives. Employees who participate in wellness activities often are offered a reduction in their insurance costs.

In keeping with a growing emphasis on value in U.S. health care, some researchers have argued that cost savings are the wrong goal for preventive health care efforts, and what should be considered is the value of the health benefits alone [229]. From this perspective, employer-based health promotion and disease prevention initiatives can provide value by improving lives at a relatively low cost and may provide a better return on investment than treatment. These costs may be outweighed by employer gains in increased productivity, decreased absenteeism, decreased staff turnover, and a healthier workforce [229].

Employers need to be included in the debates regarding the economic benefits of prevention because they have the ability to influence the environments in which adults spend large portions of their time. They also have reasons to keep their workers healthy—both to keep productivity high and to reduce the utilization of employer-provided health insurance—and can create incentives for employees to participate in wellness programs or achieve specific health indicators by tying these to reductions in the employee's health insurance premium costs.

In 2012, 63% of companies with three or more employees that offered health benefits also offered at least one wellness program [230]. Unfortunately, despite this widespread popularity, there is limited evidence regarding the effectiveness of these workplace-based wellness interventions, but the existing evidence suggests modest benefit [228]. Part of the problem with evaluating these programs is the heterogeneity of wellness initiatives across employers, which makes it difficult to aggregate results. Other problems relate to the poor quality of the research designs that seek to evaluate the effects of such programs [228]. More rigorous evaluations are needed, not only of the health effects, but also of how they translate through increased productivity and less frequent health care utilization into a return on investment for employers. Meanwhile, these programs are expected to continue to assume a greater role in the efforts of payers to manage preventable health care costs while reflecting the overall shift in U.S. health care toward wellness, disease prevention, and enhanced patient responsibility for health behavior and outcomes. BSWQA has learned that integration of employer based health risk appraisals, biometric screenings, health coaching, and wellness activities into the care model of the ACO produces continuity of care and better outcomes. Plan design by *accountable* payers and employers working with BSWQA is facilitating those results.

Conclusion

In BSWQA, we envision and are building a very different future state for Mr. B, described below:

Late in November, Mr. B is sitting at his desk looking over a memo from the human resources department. The company is offering a new health insurance plan with BSWQA as its preferred network. He notes that his out-of-pocket costs will be significantly lower if he chooses that plan, and he decides to select that option. A few days later, he is surprised to receive a call from the Member Solutions Center at BSWQA. The representative encourages him to complete a health risk assessment online and offers a convenient worksite blood draw for his biometric testing. Additionally, the representative offers and schedules an appointment with a PCP near his home. The caller concludes by suggesting that Mr. B download a suite of BSWH apps that have a variety of functions, including the ability to navigate and communicate with BSWQA providers and hospitals, plus a wealth of disease-specific information. He is impressed with the ease of this first contact.

Mr. B's previous medical history has been complicated. He is overweight and has type 2 diabetes, some type of lung problem that causes him shortness of breath, and a history of chest pains that a cardiologist has described as "stable angina." He and his wife frequently worry that he will have a major heart attack. He is supposed to take a regular aspirin and a cholesterol drug, but has been hesitant to take the cholesterol drug due to worrisome potential side effects described on the handouts from the pharmacy. Although he has tried to keep track of his visits and advice from multiple physicians, he knows that they don't communicate, because he has to relay the information over and over when he visits the cardiologist, endocrinologist, and pulmonary doctor that he sees. He has never had a relationship with a PCP other than occassional visits for minor complaints.

At his first PCP visit, he is surprised to find that he is fully preregistered. A medical assistant greets him and orients him to the entire care team, including a nurse practitioner, care coordinator, and physician. The clinic offers extended hours, video visits, and a very easy-to-use patient portal. A thorough history and exam are performed by his physician, and a comprehensive care plan for his diabetes, lung problem, and coronary disease is created. While in the PCP office, a brief three-way video visit with the cardiologist assures him that the two physicians are "on the same page" with his care plan. All of his preventive services are completed, including the flu shot he missed in September. His visit concludes with a lengthy RN care coordinator visit, where diabetes education is scheduled and his medications are again explained, giving him renewed confidence that he can actually improve his health.

Shortly after this visit, a more severe episode of chest pain causes Mr. B to drive to the nearest BSWH hospital—an "in-network" facility on his health plan. During his intake, the ED staff notes

that all of his ambulatory records are viewable
because the hospital and PCP EHR are the same.
Quick assessment reveals that a heart attack is actually occurring and the team springs into action.
A catheterization is done and a stent is placed within
30 minutes of his arrival, much better than the
national performance average. He is informed that
his damage was minimal due to the quick response.

As he nears discharge, the RN care coordinator
from his PCP office contacts him while in the hospital,
reconciling and explaining his medications, and
schedules prompt follow-up appointments for the
cardiologist and PCP.

A diabetes educator who comes to the PCP office
once weekly helps Mr. B gain understanding of his
disease and skill in administration of his insulin,
and helps him to understand blood pressure and
cholesterol goals. A mild exercise program is recommended, one that allows him to walk at work during
his lunch hour.

Mr. B's holistic and accountable care team
routinely monitors him and enables him to achieve
a much better health picture, avoiding fragmented,
redundant treatment, and encouraging engagement
in his own self-care.

This ideal scenario for Mr. B is possible through a system
of *accountable* care.

The Triple Aim challenges health care providers and
other stakeholders to improve the U.S. health care system by
enhancing the patient experience of care, improving the health
of populations, and reducing the per capita cost of health care.
Through the attainment of these goals, unsustainable rises
in health care costs may be attenuated even as high-quality
health care is delivered. As Berwick et al. wrote when
defining the Triple Aim, "Preconditions for this include the

enrollment of an identified population, a commitment to universality for its members, and the existence of an organization (an 'integrator') that accepts accountability and responsibility for all three aims for that population" [1]. The ACO movement was subsequently launched in recognition of the need for a specific organization to be accountable for the Triple Aim with respect to a defined population of patients.

This book has described both the general challenges inherent in forming, sustaining, and financing an ACO and specific experiences and lessons learned from BSWQA, which has endeavored since its founding in 2011 to bring together both independent and employed physicians, hospitals, and post–acute care and other entities along the continuum of care in an alliance with the mission of delivering the highest-quality, most cost-effective, and most coordinated care to the populations served. The book has discussed the reasons for formalizing a commitment to accountability through the creation of an ACO and has outlined the steps an ACO needs to take throughout its development, from initial organization and meeting of requirements and regulations, to the adoption of quality metrics and programs for shared financial savings, to the establishment of HIT infrastructure to drive data collection and analysis, as well as to enhance care coordination. Throughout this book, the ability to effectively manage the health of an entire population of patients has been emphasized as a key element of an ACO's commitment to *accountability*, with critical success factors for population health management including evidence-based protocols, access to affordable care, disease management, preventive health services, and strong primary care based in the PCMH model.

Achieving the Triple Aim requires a commitment to accountability not only from the physicians and hospitals constituting ACOs, but also from other stakeholders in the health care system, including providers, payers, policy makers, patients, employers, communities, and companies such as pharmaceutical manufacturers and device makers. One major challenge in driving this widespread accountability for health outcomes is that the fee-for-service payment model long predominant in the United States tends to reward volume of services provided rather than value of care delivered over time and across disparate care settings. Many have asked whether ACOs can succeed, and even whether or not health care reform can really occur with changes in the payment mechanism that rewards value over volume. Although ACOs play an important role in facilitating the adoption of value-based care and value-based payment mechanisms, the long-term success of these organizations will depend on a corresponding shift in mindset of physicians and hospital leaders to one that prioritizes high-value health outcomes at every point in the care continuum.

Notwithstanding the successes achieved by BSWQA described in this book, the future of ACOs remains uncertain. Early data are encouraging, but longer-term data are needed before robust conclusions about these organizations' sustainability can be drawn. Larger numbers of covered lives drawn into the ACO model will increase organizational attention of both physicians and hospitals as they contend with value-based reimbursements, and will require ambidextrous leadership. In the interim, quality will improve and care will become more integrated, which for patients like Mr. B is a great step forward.

In final analysis, what will determine success for ACOs? Deeply committed leadership, clear articulation of vision, and steadfast and visionary governance are fundamental. A sustained financial commitment to fund organizational structure, HIT, analytics, legal guidance, primary care and PCMH foundations, communication strategy, patient engagement, specialist engagement, hospital engagement, care coordination, wellness initiatives, and network maintenance are all requirements. New sources of value-based financing and payment changes must be negotiated. The organization will need to develop skills and processes to take on financial risk. But of all these factors, clinical and administrative leadership remains a cornerstone for success. Those leaders must daily remind physicians and hospitals of the call to professionalism, the call to *accountability* on behalf of patients, even at the disruption of current models. Their leadership call must be heard down to the provider level, for providers ultimately control both quality improvement practices and the cost of care. Primarily, the long-term success of ACOs will depend on greater provider participation and performance, but also upon the willingness of other stakeholders in the health care ecosystem to hold themselves *accountable* for the role they play in improving health and health care. This widespread assumption of responsibility will be required to drive a sustained focus on and commitment to improvement in long-term health outcomes and reduction in non-value-added cost during every care encounter. By emphasizing and encouraging accountability and the delivery of value-based care, ACOs like BSWQA are expected to continue to lead national efforts to enhance the patient experience of care, improve the health of populations, and reduce the per capita cost of health care. Accountable care organizations *can* transform care in the United States.

More important for the thousands of patients like Mr. B, substantial transformation in care delivery can be life changing. For him and others like him, we believe that personal and organizational *accountability* can and must achieve those goals.

Glossary

ABC	Accelerating Best Care
ACA	Affordable Care Act
ACO	Accountable care organization
AKS	Anti-kickback statute
BC	Best care
BHCS	Baylor Health Care System
BSWH	Baylor Scott & White Health
BSWQA	Baylor Scott & White Quality Alliance
CCD	Continuity of care document
CCHIT	Certification Commission for Healthcare Information Technology
CDA	Clinical document architecture
CDC	Centers for Disease Control and Prevention
CI	Clinical integration
CLABSI	Central-line-associated bloodstream infection
CMA	Certified medical assistant
CME	Continuing medical education
CMP	Civil monetary penalties
CMS	Centers for Medicare and Medicaid Services
COPD	Chronic obstructive pulmonary disease
CT	Computed tomography
DOJ	Department of Justice
EBM	Evidence-based medicine
ED	Emergency department

EHR	Electronic health record
FTC	Federal Trade Commission
HCC	Hierarchical condition category
HIE	Health information exchange
HIT	Health information technology
HTPN	HealthTexas Physician Network
ICU	Intensive care unit
IDN	Integrated delivery network
IHI	Institute for Healthcare Improvement
IOM	Institute of Medicine
IRS	Internal Revenue Service
IT	Information technology
LTAC	Long-term acute care
MA	Medicare Advantage
MSSP	Medicare Shared Savings Program
MRI	Magnetic resonance imaging
NCQA	National Committee on Quality Assurance
OIG	Office of the Inspector General
PCMH	Patient-centered medical home
PCP	Primary care physician
PHO	Physician-hospital organization
RAF	Risk adjustment factor
RN	Registered nurse
SOA	Service-oriented architecture
SNF	Skilled nursing facility
STEEEP	Safe, timely, effective, efficient, equitable, patient centered
SWH	Scott & White Healthcare
TIN	Tax identification number
VBP	Value-based purchasing

References

1. Berwick, D.M., T.W. Nolan, and J. Whittington. The Triple Aim: care, health, and cost. *Health Aff* (Millwood), 2008; 27(3): 759–69.
2. Institute for Healthcare Improvement. IHI Triple Aim initiative. Available from http://www.ihi.org/Engage/Initiatives/TripleAim/pages/default.aspx (cited June 10, 2015).
3. Couch, C.E., F.D. Winter Jr., and W.L. Roberts. Engaging STEEEP care through an accountable care organization. In *Achieving STEEEP Health Care*, ed. D.J. Ballard et al. Boca Raton, FL: CRC Press, 2013, 217–226.
4. The incumbent's dilemma: why disrupting yourself is hard. Available from http://rishidean.com/2014/12/08/incumbents-dilemma-why-disrupting-yourself-is-hard/ ().
5. National Committee on Quality Assurance. Patient-centered medical home recognition. Available from http://www.ncqa.org/Programs/Recognition/Practices/PatientCenteredMedicalHomePCMH.aspx (cited June 17, 2015).
6. Bodenheimer, T. Coordinating care—a perilous journey through the health care system. *N Engl J Med*, 2008; 358(10): 1064–71.
7. Corrigan, J.M., M.S. Donaldson, L.T. Kohn, S.K. Maguire, and K.C. Pike. *Crossing the Quality Chasm: A New Health System for the 21st Century*. Washington, DC: National Academy Press, 2001.
8. Agency for Healthcare Research and Quality. The number of practicing primary care physicians in the United States. Available from http://www.ahrq.gov/research/findings/factsheets/primary/pcwork1/ (cited July 2, 2015).

9. Bernstein, L. Once again, U.S. has most expensive, least effective health care system in survey. Washington Post, June 16, 2014. Available from http://www.washingtonpost.com/news/to-your-health/wp/2014/06/16/once-again-u-s-has-most-expensive-least-effective-health-care-system-in-survey/ (cited June 10, 2015).

10. Woolf, S.H., and L.Y. Aron. The US health disadvantage relative to other high-income countries: findings from a National Research Council/Institute of Medicine report. *JAMA*, 2013; 309(8): 771–72.

11. Berwick, D.M., and A.D. Hackbarth. Eliminating waste in US health care. *JAMA*, 2012; 307(14): 1513–16.

12. Fisher, E.S., et al. Creating accountable care organizations: the extended hospital medical staff. *Health Aff* (Millwood), 2007; 26(1): w44–57.

13. Health Affairs. Health policy briefs: next steps for ACOs. Available from http://www.healthaffairs.org/healthpolicybriefs/brief.php?brief_id=61 (cited June 10, 2015).

14. Patient Protection and Affordable Care Act. 2010.

15. Health Affairs Blog. Growth and dispersion of accountable care organizations in 2015. March 21, 2015. Available from http://healthaffairs.org/blog/2015/03/31/growth-and-dispersion-of-accountable-care-organizations-in-2015-2/ (cited June 10, 2015).

16. American Hospital Association. Trendwatch clinical integration: the key to real reform. American Hospital Association, February 2010. Chicago, IL.

17. Rittenhouse, D.R., S.M. Shortell, and E.S. Fisher. Primary care and accountable care—two essential elements of delivery-system reform. *N Engl J Med*, 2009; 361(24): 2301–3.

18. NOVA. The Hippocratic Oath today. Available from http://www.pbs.org/wgbh/nova/body/hippocratic-oath-today.html (cited June 10, 2015).

19. Porter, M.E. What is value in health care? *N Engl J Med*, 2010; 363(26): 2477–81.

20. Merriam-Webster. Accountability. Available from http://www.merriam-webster.com/dictionary/accountability (cited June 10, 2015).

21. Partners for Health Reform*plus*. Accountability and health systems: overview, framework, and strategies. Available from http://www.who.int/management/partnerships/accountability/AccountabilityHealthSystemsOverview.pdf (cited June 10, 2015).

22. Gamm, L.D. Dimensions of accountability for not-for-profit hospitals and health systems. *Health Care Manage Rev*, 1996; 21(2): 74–86.
23. McGlynn, E.A., et al. The quality of health care delivered to adults in the United States. *N Engl J Med*, 2003; 348(26): 2635–45.
24. Kohn, L.T., J.M. Corrigan, and M.S. Donaldson, eds. *To Err Is Human: Building a Safer Health System: A Report from the Committee on Quality of Healthcare in America.* Washington, DC: National Academy Press, Institute of Medicine, National Academy of Sciences, 1999.
25. Boudreau, R.M., et al. Improving the timeliness of written patient notification of mammography results by mammography centers. *Breast J*, 2004; 10(1): 10–19.
26. Kwan, J., P. Hand, and P. Sandercock. Improving the efficiency of delivery of thrombolysis for acute stroke: a systematic review. *QJM*, 2004; 97(5): 273–79.
27. Himelhoch, S., et al. Chronic medical illness, depression, and use of acute medical services among Medicare beneficiaries. *Med Care*, 2004; 42(6): 512–21.
28. Anderson, G., and J. Horvath. Chronic conditions: making the case for ongoing care. 2002. Available from http://www.partnershipforsolutions.org/DMS/files/chronicbook2002.pdf (cited June 10, 2015).
29. Sepucha, K., and A.G. Mulley Jr. A perspective on the patient's role in treatment decisions. *Med Care Res Rev*, 2009; 66(1 Suppl): 53S–74S.
30. Braddock, C.H., 3rd, et al. Informed decision making in out-patient practice: time to get back to basics. *JAMA*, 1999; 282(24): 2313–20.
31. Dentzer, S. Still crossing the quality chasm–or suspended over it? *Health Aff* (Millwood), 2011; 30(4): 554–55.
32. Modern Healthcare. About that quality chasm. Available from http://www.modernhealthcare.com/article/20110221/MAGAZINE/110219950 (cited June 10, 2015).
33. Ballard, D.J., et al. Improving delivery of clinical preventive services: a multi-year journey. *Am J Prev Med*, 2007; 33(6): 492–97.
34. Ballard, D.J., et al. *Achieving STEEEP Health Care.* Boca Raton, FL: CRC Press, 2013.
35. Silverstein, M.D., et al. Impact of clinical preventive services in the ambulatory setting. *Proc* (Bayl Univ Med Cent), 2008; 21(3): 227–35.

36. National Committee on Quality Assurance. HEDIS & performance measurement. Available from http://www.ncqa.org/HEDISQualityMeasurement.aspx (cited June 10, 2015).

37. Bureau of Labor Statistics. Databases, tables & calculators by subject. Available from http://data.bls.gov/ (cited June 10, 2015).

38. Hussey, P.S., et al. Controlling U.S. health care spending—separating promising from unpromising approaches. *N Engl J Med*, 2009; 361(22): 2109–11.

39. Gawande, A.A., et al. The cost of health care—highlights from a discussion about economics and reform. *N Engl J Med*, 2009; 361(15): 1421–23.

40. Kaplan, R.S., and M.E. Porter. The big idea: how to solve the cost crisis in health care. *Harv Bus Rev*, 2011; 89(9): 46–52, 54, 56–61.

41. Squires, D.A. *Explaining High Health Care Spending in the United States: An International Comparison of Supply, Utilization, Prices, and Quality.* New York: The Commonwealth Fund, 2012.

42. The World Bank. Health expenditure per capita. Available from http://data.worldbank.org/indicator/SH.XPD.PCAP (cited February 10, 2014).

43. Finkelstein, E.A., et al. Annual medical spending attributable to obesity: payer-and service-specific estimates. *Health Aff* (Millwood), 2009; 28(5): w822–31.

44. International Federation of Health Plans (IFHP). *Comparative Price Report: Medical and Hospital Fees by Country.* London: IFHP, 2011.

45. Laugesen, M.J., and S.A. Glied. Higher fees paid to US physicians drive higher spending for physician services compared to other countries. *Health Aff* (Millwood), 2011; 30(9): 1647–56.

46. Averill, R.F., N. Goldfield, and J.S. Hughes. Distributing shared savings for population health management. *Healthc Financ Manage*, 2014; 68(4): 46–49.

47. Berwick, D.M. Launching accountable care organizations—the proposed rule for the Medicare Shared Savings Program. *N Engl J Med*, 2011; 364(16): e32.

48. Schedler, A. Conceptualizing accountability. In *The Self-Restraining State: Power and Accountability in New Democracies*, ed. A. Schedler, L. Diamond, and M.F. Plattner. Boulder, CO: Lynne Rienner Publishers, 1999, 13–29.

49. Peterson, M., and D. Muhlestein. ACO Results: what we know so far. Health Affairs Blog. Available from http://healthaffairs.org/blog/2014/05/30/aco-results-what-we-know-so-far/ (cited June 11, 2015).

50. ACO toolkit: accountable care learning network. 2011. Available from https://xteam.brookings.edu/bdacoln/Documents/ACO%20Toolkit%20January%202011.pdf (cited May 28, 2015).

51. Medical Device and Diagnostic Industry. ACO hospital model will influence medical device makers. Available from http://www.mddionline.com/blog/devicetalk/aco-hospital-model-will-influence-medical-device-makers (cited June 11, 2015).

52. Noble, D.J., T. Greenhalgh, and L.P. Casalino. Improving population health one person at a time? Accountable care organisations: perceptions of population health—a qualitative interview study. *BMJ Open*, 2014; 4(4): e004665.

53. Muhlestein, D.B., A.A. Croshaw, and T.P. Merrill. Risk bearing and use of fee-for-service billing among accountable care organizations. *Am J Manag Care*, 2013; 19(7): 589–92.

54. Musich, S., et al. An evaluation of the Well at Dell health management program: health risk change and financial return on investment. *Am J Health Promot*, 2015; 29(3): 147–57.

55. Devore, S., and R.W. Champion. Driving population health through accountable care organizations. *Health Aff* (Millwood), 2011; 30(1): 41–50.

56. Camargo, R., et al. Accountable care organizations: financial advantages of larger hospital organizations. *Health Care Manag* (Frederick), 2014; 33(2): 110–16.

57. L&M Policy Research. Evaluation of CMMI accountable care organization initiatives. Available from http://innovation.cms.gov/Files/reports/PioneerACOEvalReport1.pdf (cited June 11, 2015).

58. Barnes, A.J., et al. Accountable care organizations in the USA: types, developments and challenges. *Health Policy*, 2014; 118(1): 1–7.

59. Koury, C., et al. The accountable care organization summit: a white paper on findings, outcomes, and challenges. *Hosp Top*, 2014; 92(2): 44–57.

60. Ortolon, K. The Texas twist. *Tex Med*, 2011; 107(9): 31–33.

61. Muhlestein, D., et al. *Growth and Dispersion of Accountable Care Organizations: June 2012 Update*. Washington, DC: Leavitt Partners, 2012.

62. Muhlestein, D., et al. A taxonomy of accountable care organizations: different approached to achieve the Triple Aim. 2014. Available from http://www.leavittpartners.com/wp-content/uploads/2014/06/A-Taxonomy-of-Accountable-Care-Organizations.pdf (cited May 28, 2015).

63. Colla, C.H., et al. First national survey of ACOs finds that physicians are playing strong leadership and ownership roles. *Health Aff* (Millwood), 2014; 33(6): 964–71.

64. Shortell, S.M., et al. A taxonomy of accountable care organizations for policy and practice. *Health Serv Res*, 2014; 49(6): 1883–99.

65. Kocher, R., and N.R. Sahni. Physicians versus hospitals as leaders of accountable care organizations. *N Engl J Med*, 2010; 363(27): 2579–82.

66. Tilburt, J.C., et al. Views of US physicians about controlling health care costs. *JAMA*, 2013; 310(4): 380–88.

67. Shields, M. From clinical integration to accountable care. *Ann Health Law*, 2011; 20(2): 151–64.

68. Terry, K. Health IT: the glue for accountable care organizations. Four big systems show how they're using EHRs, connectivity, and data warehouses to drive ACOs. Healthc Inform, 2011; 28(5): 16, 18, 20 passim.

69. Couch, C.E., F.D. Winter Jr., and W.L. Roberts. Driving STEEEP care across a physician provider network. In *Achieving STEEEP Health Care*, ed. D.J. Ballard et al. Boca Raton, FL: CRC Press, 2013, 99–112.

70. Herrin, J., D. Nicewander, and D.J. Ballard. The effect of health care system administrator pay-for-performance on quality of care. *Jt Comm J Qual Patient Saf*, 2008; 34(11): 646–54.

71. Kennerly, D., et al. STEEEP analytics. In *Achieving STEEEP Health Care*, ed. D.J. Ballard et al. Boca Raton, FL: CRC Press, 2013, 75–80.

72. Fullerton, C., J. Sullivan, and B. da Graca. One ACO's journey to comprehensive–connected–continuous care. In *Population Health: An Implementation Guide to Improve Outcomes and Lower Costs*, ed. G. Mayzell. New York: Productivity Press, 2015.

73. Moore, K.D., and D.C. Coddington. *The Work Ahead: Activities and Costs to Develop an Accountable Care Organization*. Chicago: American Hospital Association, 2011.

74. Sandberg, S.F., et al. Hennepin Health: a safety-net accountable care organization for the expanded Medicaid population. *Health Aff* (Millwood), 2014; 33(11): 1975–84.

75. Association of American Medical Colleges. Physician supply and demand through 2025: key findings. 2015. Available from https://www.aamc.org/download/426260/data/physiciansupply anddemandthrough2025keyfindings.pdf (cited June 2015).

76. HIMSS. Health information exhange. Available from http://www.himss.org/library/health-information-exchange?navItem Number=16135 (cited May 15, 2015).

77. Texas Tribune. Interactive: mapping access to health care in Texas. May 8, 2012. Available from http://www.texastribune. org/library/data/texas-shortage-health-care-providers/?%20 utm_source=texastribune.org&utm_medium=alerts&utm_ campaign=News%20Alert:%20Subscriptions (cited June 28, 2015).

78. Chandra, A., M.A. Dalton, and J. Holmes. Large increases in spending on postacute care in Medicare point to the potential for cost savings in these settings. *Health Aff* (Millwood), 2013; 32(5): 864–72.

79. *Health Care Fraud: Types of Providers Involved in Medicare, Medicaid, and the Children's Health Insurance Program Cases.* Washington, DC: U.S. Government Accountability Office, 2012.

80. O'Malley, A.S., A.M. Bond, and R.A. Berenson. Rising hospital employment of physicians: better quality, higher costs? 2011. Available from http://www.hschange.com/CONTENT/1230/ (cited June 1, 2015).

81. Naylor, M.D., and E.T. Kurtzman. The role of nurse practitioners in reinventing primary care. *Health Aff* (Millwood), 2010; 29(5): 893–99.

82. 42 CFR § 411.357(w).

83. 42 CFR § 1001.952(y).

84. Baylor Scott & White Quality Alliance (BSWQA). Value report. BSWQA, 2014. Dallas, TX.

85. Brook, R.H. Why not big ideas and big interventions? *J Gen Intern Med*, 2014; 29(12): 1586–88.

86. Toussaint, J., A. Milstein, and S. Shortell. How the Pioneer ACO model needs to change: lessons from its best-performing ACO. *JAMA*, 2013; 310(13): 1341–42.

87. Department of Health and Human Services. Better, smarter, healthier: in historic announcement, HHS sets clear goals and timeline for shifting Medicare reimbursements from volume to value. 2015. Available from http://www.hhs.gov/news/ press/2015pres/01/20150126a.html (cited June 16, 2015).

88. Lineen, J. Hospital consolidation: "safety in numbers" strategy prevails in preparation for a value-based marketplace. *J Healthc Manag*, 2014; 59(5): 315–17.

89. Friedburg, M.W., et al. *Effects of Health Care Payment Models on Physician Practice in the United States.* Santa Monica, CA: RAND Corporation, 2015

90. Postma, J., and A.F. Roos. Why healthcare providers merge. *Health Econ Policy Law*, 2015; 1–20.

91. *Arizona v. Maricopa County Medical Society.* 1982, 457 U.S. 332.

92. Department of Justice and Federal Trade Commission. Statements of antitrust enforcement policy in health care. 1996. Available from http://www.justice.gov/atr/public/guidelines/0000.htm (cited June 12, 2015).

93. Federal Trade Commission and Department of Justice. Statement of antitrust enforcement policy regarding accountable care organizations participating in the Medicare Shared Savings Program. 76 *Fed Reg* 67026–67031 (October 28, 2011).

94. Federal Trade Commission. Follow-up to 2002 Medsouth, Inc. staff advisory opinion. 2007. Available from www.ftc.gov/sites/default/files/documents/advisory-opinions/medsouth-inc./070618medsouth.pdf (cited June 29, 2015).

95. Dallas Business Journal. DFW ACOs, who are the local dance partners? 2013. Available from http://www.bizjournals.com/dallas/print-edition/2013/02/22/dfw-acos-who-are-the-local-dance.html (cited June 12, 2015).

96. 42 USC § 1395jjj.

97 Department of Health and Human Services, Medicare Program. Medicare Shared Savings Program: accountable care organizations. 76 *Fed Reg* 67802–67990 (November 2, 2011).

98. Couch, C.E. Why Baylor Health Care System would like to file for Medicare Shared Savings accountable care organization designation but cannot. *Mayo Clin Proc*, 2012; 87(8): 723–26.

99. 42 USC § 1320a-7b(b).

100. *Redlands Surgical Servs. v. Commissioner of Internal Revenue.* 1999, U.S. Tax Court 47.

101. *St. David's Health Care System v. United States.* 2003, 5th Cir. 232.

102. 42 CFR § 1001.952.

103. Department of Health and Human Services and Office of the Inspector General, Medicare and State Health Care Programs. Fraud and abuse; safe harbors for protecting health plans. 61 *Fed Reg* 2122, 2123 (January 25, 1996).

104. 42 USC § 1320a-7b(b)(3)(B).

105. 42 CFR § 1001.952(d), (i).

106. 42 USC § 1395nn.

107. 42 USC § 1395nn(e)(2)–(3).

108. 42 CFR § 411.357(c), (d).

109. 42 CFR § 411.351.

110. 42 USC § 1320a-7a(b).

111. Office of the Inspector General. Gainsharing arrangements and CMPs for hospital payments to physicians to reduce or limit services to beneficiaries. 1999. Available from http://oig.hhs.gov/fraud/docs/alertsandbulletins/gainsh.htm (cited June 12, 2015).

112. Department of Health and Human Services and Office of the Inspector General. OIG Advisory Opinion No. 08-21. 2008. Available from https://oig.hhs.gov/fraud/docs/advisoryopinions/2008/AdvOpn08–21.2.pdf (cited June 12, 2015).

113. Medicare Access and CHIP Reauthorization Act, Pub. L. No. 114-10. 2015.

114. Department of Health and Human Services, Centers for Medicare and Medicaid Services, and Office of the Inspector General, Medicare Program. Final waivers in connection with the Shared Savings Program. 76 *Fed Reg* 67991–68010 (November 2, 2011).

115. Homchick, R.G., and S. Fallows. ACOs: fraud & abuse waivers and analysis. Available from https://www.healthlawyers.org/events/programs/materials/documents/hct13/h_homchick.pdf (cited June 12, 2015).

116. 26 CFR 1.501(c)(3)–1(c)(2).

117. 26 CFR 1.501(c)(3)–1(d)(1)(ii).

118. Internal Revenue Service. Notice 2011–20. 2011. Available from http://www.irs.gov/pub/irs-drop/n-11–20.pdf (cited June 12, 2015).

119. Pearl, R. True physician leadership key to sustainability of ACOs. *Mod Healthc*, 2014; 44(49): 27.

120. Tjosvold, D., and R.C. MacPherson. Joint hospital management by physicians and nursing administrators. *Health Care Manage Rev*, 1996; 21(3): 43–54.

121. Porter, M.E., and E.O. Teisberg. *Redefining Health Care: Creating Value-Based Competition on Results*. Boston: Harvard Business Press, 2006.

122. Swensen, S.J., et al. Controlling healthcare costs by removing waste: what American doctors can do now. *BMJ Qual Saf*, 2011; 20(6): 534–37.

123. Goeschel, C.A., R.M. Wachter, and P.J. Pronovost. Responsibility for quality improvement and patient safety: hospital board and medical staff leadership challenges. *Chest*, 2010; 138(1): 171–78.

124. Convery, P., C.E. Couch, and R. Luquire. Training physician and nursing leaders for performance improvement. In *From Front Office to Front Line: Essential Issues for Health Care Leaders*. Oakbrook Terrace, IL: Joint Commission Resources, 2012, 59–86.

125. Stoller, J.K. Developing physician-leaders: key competencies and available programs. *J Health Adm Educ*, 2008; 25(4): 307–28.

126. Stoller, J.K. Developing physician-leaders: a call to action. *J Gen Intern Med*, 2009; 24(7): 876–78.

127. Baylor Scott & White Quality Alliance. Leadership. Available from http://www.baylorqualityalliance.com/leadership/Pages/leadership.aspx (cited January 19, 2015).

128. Sackett, D., et al. *Evidence-Based Medicine: How to Practise and Teach EBM*, 2nd ed. Edinburgh: Churchill-Livingstone, 2000.

129. Wennberg, J. Time to tackle unwarranted variations in practice. *BMJ*, 2011; 342: d1513.

130. Ballard, D.J., B. da Graca, and D. Nicewander. Variations in care. In *Medical Epidemiology: Population Health and Effective Health Care*, ed. R.S. Greenberg. New York: McGraw-Hill Education, 2015.

131. Sadeghi-Bazargani, H., J.S. Tabrizi, and S. Azami-Aghdash. Barriers to evidence-based medicine: a systematic review. *J Eval Clin Pract*, 2014; 20(6): 793–802.

132. Ruokoniemi, P., et al. Are statin trials in diabetes representative of real-world diabetes care: a population-based study on statin initiators in Finland. *BMJ Open*, 2014; 4(6): e005402.

133. Bartlett, C., et al. The causes and effects of socio-demographic exclusions from clinical trials. *Health Technol Assess*, 2005; 9(38): iii–iv, ix–x, 1–152.

134. Morris, Z.S., S. Wooding, and J. Grant. The answer is 17 years, what is the question: understanding time lags in translational research. *J R Soc Med, 2011*; 104(12): 510–20.

135. Zwolsman, S., et al. Barriers to GPs' use of evidence-based medicine: a systematic review. *Br J Gen Pract*, 2012; 62(600): e511–21.

136. Cochrane: about us. Available from http://www.cochrane.org/about-us (cited June 1, 2015).

137. Mostofian, F., et al. Changing physician behavior: what works? *Am J Manag Care*, 2015; 21(1): 75–84.

138. National Quality Forum. 0092 emergency medicine: aspirin at arrival for acute myocardial infarction (AMI). Available from http://www.qualityforum.org/Qps/QpsTool.aspx (cited June 25, 2015).

139. Centers for Disease Control and Prevention. Hand hygiene in healthcare settings. Available from http://www.cdc.gov/handhygiene/Guidelines.html (cited June 25, 2015).

140. US Preventive Services Task Force. Published recommendations. Available from http://www.uspreventiveservicestaskforce.org/BrowseRec/Index/browse-recommendations (cited June 25, 2015).

141. ABIM Foundation. Choosing Wisely®. Available from http://www.choosingwisely.org/ (cited May 15, 2013).

142. Ballard, D.J., B. da Graca, and D. Nicewander. Quality of care. In *Medical Epidemiology: Population Health and Effective Health Care*, ed. R.S. Greenberg. New York: McGraw-Hill Education, 2015.

143. McClellan, M.B., S.L. Kocot, and R. White. Early evidence on Medicare ACOs and next steps for the Medicare ACO program (updated). 2015. Available from http://healthaffairs.org/blog/2015/01/22/early-evidence-on-medicare-acos-and-next-steps-for-the-medicare-aco-program/ (cited June 1, 2015).

144. Kocot, S.L., et al. A more complete picture of Pioneer ACO results. 2014. Available from http://www.brookings.edu/blogs/up-front/posts/2014/10/09-pioneer-aco-results-mcclellan#recent_rr/ (cited June 1, 2015).

145. Burns, L.R., and M.V. Pauly. Accountable care organizations may have difficulty avoiding the failures of integrated delivery networks of the 1990s. *Health Aff* (Millwood), 2012; 31(11): 2407–16.

146. Casalino, L.P. Accountable care organizations—the risk of failure and the risks of success. *N Engl J Med*, 2014; 371(18): 1750–51.

147. Colla, C.H., and E.S. Fisher. Beyond PCMHs and accountable care organizations: payment reform that encourages customized care. *J Gen Intern Med*, 2014; 29(10): 1325–27.

148. Christensen, C., J. Flier, and V. Vijayaraghavan. The coming failure of 'accountable care.' 2013. Available from http://www.wsj.com/articles/SB10001424127887324880504578296902005944398 (cited June 1, 2015).

149. Weeks, W.B., et al. Higher health care quality and bigger savings found at large multispecialty medical groups. *Health Aff* (Millwood), 2010; 29(5): 991–97.

150. Council of Accountable Physician Practices. Why are account-able care organizations important to achieve improved cost and quality? Available from http://www.accountablecarefacts.org/topten/why-is-health-care-delivery-reform-as-proposed-in-the-affordable-care-act-necessary-1 (cited June 1, 2015).

151. Crosson, F.J. Analysis & commentary: the accountable care orga-nization: whatever its growing pains, the concept is too vitally important to fail. *Health Aff* (Millwood), 2011; 30(7): 1250–55.

152. Khullar, D., et al. Behavioral economics and physician compen-sation—promise and challenges. *N Engl J Med*, 2015; 372(24): 2281–83.

153. Cohen, S.B., et al. Increasing consumerism in healthcare through intelligent information technology. *Am J Manag Care*, 2010; 16(12 Suppl HIT): SP37–43.

154. Robinson, J.C. Managed consumerism in health care. *Health Aff* (Millwood), 2005; 24(6): 1478–89.

155. Arnold, S.B. improving quality health care: the role of consumer engagement. Available from http://www.academyhealth.org/files/issues/ConsumerEngagement.pdf (cited May 4, 2015).

156. Hibbard, J.H., and J. Greene. What the evidence shows about patient activation: better health outcomes and care experiences; fewer data on costs. *Health Aff* (Millwood), 2013; 32(2): 207–14.

157. Greene, J., et al. When patient activation levels change, health outcomes and costs change, too. *Health Aff* (Millwood), 2015; 34(3): 431–37.

158. Mitchell, S.E., et al. Patient activation and 30-day post-discharge hospital utilization. *J Gen Intern Med*, 2014; 29(2): 349–55.

159. Fowles, J.B., et al. Measuring self-management of patients' and employees' health: further validation of the Patient Activation Measure (PAM) based on its relation to employee characteris-tics. *Patient Educ Couns*, 2009; 77(1): 116–22.

160. Robinson, J.C., and T.T. Brown. Increases in consumer cost sharing redirect patient volumes and reduce hospital prices for orthopedic surgery. *Health Aff* (Millwood), 2013; 32(8): 1392–97.

161. Zimmer, B. Wellness. *New York Times Magazine*. April 18, 2010: mm20.

162. Cortez, N.G., I.G. Cohen, and A.S. Kesselheim. FDA regulation of mobile health technologies. *N Engl J Med*, 2014; 371(4): 372–79.

163. Rainie, L. Cell phone ownership hits 91% of adults. Pew Research Center, 2013, Washington, D.C.

164. de Jongh, T., et al. Mobile phone messaging for facilitating self-management of long-term illnesses. *Cochrane Database Syst Rev*, 2012; 12: CD007459.

165. Free, C., et al. The effectiveness of mobile-health technology-based health behaviour change or disease management interventions for health care consumers: a systematic review. *PLoS Med*, 2013; 10(1): e1001362.

166. Nundy, S., et al. Mobile phone diabetes project led to improved glycemic control and net savings for Chicago plan participants. *Health Aff* (Millwood), 2014; 33(2): 265–72.

167. McGillicuddy, J.W., et al. Patient attitudes toward mobile phone-based health monitoring: questionnaire study among kidney transplant recipients. *J Med Internet Res*, 2013; 15(1): e6.

168. Proudfoot, J., et al. Community attitudes to the appropriation of mobile phones for monitoring and managing depression, anxiety, and stress. *J Med Internet Res*, 2010; 12(5): e64.

169. research2guidance. research2guidance's mHealth App Developer Economics 2014. 2014. Available from: http://rhttp:// research2guidance.com/r2g/research2guidance-mHealth-App-Developer-Economics-2014.pdf (cited September 16, 2015).

170. Helm, A.M. Privacy and mHealth: how mobile health "apps" fit into a privacy framework not limited to HIPAA. *Syracuse Law Rev*, 2014; 64: 131–170.

171. Kahn, J.M. Virtual visits—confronting the challenges of tele-medicine. *N Engl J Med*, 2015; 372(18): 1684–85.

172. Adler-Milstein, J., J. Kvedar, and D.W. Bates. Telehealth among US hospitals: several factors, including state reimbursement and licensure policies, influence adoption. *Health Aff* (Millwood), 2014; 33(2): 207–15.

173. HIMSS Analytics. Essentials brief: US telemedicine study. 2014. Available from https://www.himssanalytics.org/research/essentials-brief-us-telemedicine-study (cited May 14, 2015).

174. Pearl, R. Kaiser Permanente Northern California: current experiences with Internet, mobile, and video technologies. *Health Aff* (Millwood), 2014; 33(2): 251–57.

175. Robert Wood Johnson Foundation. Retail clinics. Available from http://www.countyhealthrankings.org/policies/retail-clinics (cited May 14, 2015).
176. Shrank, W.H., et al. Quality of care at retail clinics for 3 common conditions. *Am J Manag Care*, 2014; 20(10): 794–801.
177. Jacoby, R., et al. Quality of care for 2 common pediatric conditions treated by convenient care providers. *Am J Med Qual*, 2011; 26(1): 53–58.
178. Rohrer, J.E., G.M. Garrison, and K.B. Angstman. Early return visits by pediatric primary care patients with otitis media: a retail nurse practitioner clinic versus standard medical office care. *Qual Manag Health Care*, 2012; 21(1): 44–47.
179. Sussman, A., et al. Retail clinic utilization associated with lower total cost of care. *Am J Manag Care*, 2013; 19(4): e148–57.
180. Mehrotra, A., et al. Comparing costs and quality of care at retail clinics with that of other medical settings for 3 common illnesses. *Ann Intern Med*, 2009; 151(5): 321–28.
181. Garbutt, J.M., et al. Parents' experiences with pediatric care at retail clinics. *JAMA Pediatr*, 2013; 167(9): 845–50.
182. Wang, M.C., et al. Why do patients seek care at retail clinics, and what alternatives did they consider? *Am J Med Qual*, 2010; 25(2): 128–34.
183. Modern Healthcare. Retail clinics at tipping point. Available from http://www.modernhealthcare.com/article/20130504/MAGAZINE/305049991 (cited May 14, 2015).
184. Advisory Board Company. From vaccinations to ACOs: retailers expand health care services. Available from http://www.advisory.com/daily-briefing/2013/05/08/retailers-expand-into-primary-accountable-care (cited May 14, 2015).
185. Centers for Medicare and Medicaid Services. Hospital value-based purchasing. Available from https://www.cms.gov/Medicare/Quality-Initiatives-Patient-Assessment-Instruments/hospital-value-based-purchasing/index.html?redirect=/hospital-value-based-purchasing (cited May 15, 2015).
186. Modern Healthcare. More hospitals to get bonuses than penalties in 2015 under value-based purchasing. Available from http://www.modernhealthcare.com/article/20141218/NEWS/141219982 (cited May 15, 2015).
187. Joynt, K.E., and A.K. Jha. A path forward on Medicare readmissions. *N Engl J Med*, 2013; 368(13): 1175–77.

188. LaMantia, M.A., et al. Interventions to improve transitional care between nursing homes and hospitals: a systematic review. *J Am Geriatr Soc*, 2010; 58(4): 777–82.

189. Naylor, M.D., et al. Transitional care of older adults hospitalized with heart failure: a randomized, controlled trial. *J Am Geriatr Soc*, 2004; 52(5): 675–84.

190. Peikes, D., et al. Effects of care coordination on hospitalization, quality of care, and health care expenditures among Medicare beneficiaries: 15 randomized trials. *JAMA*, 2009; 301(6): 603–18.

191. Stauffer, B.D., et al. Effectiveness and cost of a transitional care program for heart failure: a prospective study with concurrent controls. *Arch Intern Med*, 2011; 171(14): 1238–43.

192. Agency for Healthcare Research and Quality. The concentration of health care expenditures and related expenses for costly medical conditions. 2009. Available from http://meps.ahrq.gov/mepsweb/data_files/publications/st359/stat359.pdf (cited June 13, 2015).

193. Health Care Advisory Board. *Playbook for Population Health: Building the High-Performance Care Management Network.* Health Care Advisory Board, 2013, Washington, D.C.

194. Hollander, P., et al. Quality of care of Medicare patients with diabetes in a metropolitan fee-for-service primary care integrated delivery system. *Am J Med Qual*, 2005; 20(6): 344–52.

195. Herrin, J., et al. The effectiveness of implementing an electronic health record on diabetes care and outcomes. *Health Serv Res*, 2012; 47(4): 1522–40.

196. Patient-Centered Medical Home Advisory Committee. 2014. *Standards and Guidelines for NCQA's Patient-Centered Medical Home (PCMH) 2014.* Washington, D.C.: National Committee for Quality Assurance.

197. Taliani, C.A., et al. Implementing effective care management in the patient-centered medical home. Am J Manag Care, 2013; 19(12): 957–64.

198. National Quality Forum. NQF-endorsed definition and framework for measuring care coordination. Available from http://216.122.138.39/pdf/reports/ambulatory_endorsed_definition.pdf (cited January 21, 2007).

199. Huffman, M. Using motivational interviewing: through evidence-based health coaching. *Home Healthc Nurse*, 2014; 32(9): 543–48.

200. Calvillo-King, L., et al. Impact of social factors on risk of readmission or mortality in pneumonia and heart failure: systematic review. *J Gen Intern Med*, 2013; 28(2): 269–82.

201. Greysen, S.R., et al. "Missing pieces"—functional, social, and environmental barriers to recovery for vulnerable older adults transitioning from hospital to home. *J Am Geriatr Soc*, 2014; 62(8): 1556–61.

202. Centeno, M.M., and K.L. Kahveci. Transitional care models: preventing readmissions for high-risk patient populations. *Crit Care Nurs Clin North Am*, 2014; 26(4): 589–97.

203. Stutman, H. A longitudinal medical record is key to clinical decision support. Available from http://www.clinical-innovation. com/topics/ehr-emr/longitudinal-medical-record-key-clinical-decision-support (cited June 14, 2015).

204. Miller, H.D. How to create accountable care organizations. Center of Healthcare Quality & Payment Reform, September 2009, Pittsburgh, PA.

205. Hahn, H.F., and T.A. Criger. accountable care organizations: physician participation required. America Health Lawyers Association, January 2011, Washington, D.C.

206. Centers for Medicare and Medicaid Services. Press release: CMS names 89 new Medicare Shared Savings accountable care organizations. 2012. Available from https://www.cms.gov/apps/ media/press/factsheet.asp?Counter=4405&intNumPerPage=10 &checkDate=&checkKey=&srchType=1&numDays=3500&sr ch Opt=0&srchData=&keywordType=All&chkNewsTypc=6& int Page=&showAll=&pYear=&year=&desc=&cboOrder=date (cited July 9, 2012).

207. Allscripts. dbMotion. Available from http://www.allscripts.com/ products-services/products/dbmotion (cited June 14, 2015).

208. KLAS. About KLAS. Available from http://www.klasresearch. com/about/company.aspx (cited June 14, 2015).

209. Jha, A.K., et al. Measuring efficiency: the association of hospital costs and quality of care. *Health Aff* (Millwood), 2009; 28(3): 897–906.

210. Fisher, E.S., et al. The implications of regional variations in Medicare spending. Part 2: health outcomes and satisfaction with care. *Ann Intern Med*, 2003; 138(4): 288–98.

211. Gawande, A. The cost conundrum. *The New Yorker*, June 1, 2009.

212. Fisher, E.S., J.P. Bynum, and J.S. Skinner. Slowing the growth of health care costs—lessons from regional variation. *N Engl J Med*, 2009; 360(9): 849–52.

213. Colla, C.H., et al. Choosing wisely: prevalence and correlates of low-value health care services in the United States. *J Gen Intern Med*, 2015; 30(2): 221–28.

214. Sirovich, B., et al. Discretionary decision making by primary care physicians and the cost of U.S. health care. *Health Aff* (Millwood), 2008; 27(3): 813–23.

215. Centers for Disease Control and Prevention. The state of aging and health in America 2013. Available from http://www.cdc. gov/features/agingandhealth/state_of_aging_and_health_in_ america_2013.pdf (cited June 15, 2015).

216. Hoover, D.R., et al. Medical expenditures during the last year of life: findings from the 1992–1996 Medicare current beneficiary survey. *Health Serv Res*, 2002; 37(6): 1625–42.

217. HealthIT.gov. EHR incentives and certifications. Available from http://www.healthit.gov/providers-professionals/meaningful-use-definition-objectives (cited May 12, 2015).

218. Chaudhry, B., et al. Systematic review: impact of health information technology on quality, efficiency, and costs of medical care. *Ann Intern Med*, 2006; 144(10): 742–52.

219. Fleming, N.S., et al. The impact of electronic health records on workflow and financial measures in primary care practices. *Health Serv Res*, 2014; 49(1 Pt 2): 405–20.

220. Song, P.H., et al. Exploring the business case for ambulatory electronic health record system adoption. *J Healthc Manag*, 2011; 56(3): 169–80; discussion 181–82.

221. Agency for Healthcare Research and Quality. State snapshots 2011. Available from http://statesnapshots.ahrq.gov/snaps11/ (cited May 15, 2013).

222. Hardin, G. The tragedy of the commons: the population problem has no technical solution; it requires a fundamental extension in morality. *Science*, 1968; 162(3859): 1243–48.

223. de Brantes, F., M.B. Rosenthal, and M. Painter. Building a bridge from fragmentation to accountability—he Prometheus payment model. *N Engl J Med*, 2009; 361(11): 1033–36.

224. Blumenthal, D. Reflecting on health reform—narrow networks: boon or bane? Commonweath Fund Blog. Available from http://www.commonwealthfund.org/publications/blog/2014/feb/narrows-networks-boon-or-bane (cited June 18, 2015).

225. Bodenheimer, T.S., and M.D. Smith. Primary care: proposed solutions to the physician shortage without training more physicians. *Health Aff* (Millwood), 2013; 32(11): 1881–86.
226. Bluentritt, R.M., and G.D. Anderson. ACO shared savings distribution models. American Health Lawyers Association, May 2013, Washington, D.C.
227. Centers for Medicare and Medicaid Services. Comprehensive primary care initiative. Available from http://innovation.cms.gov/initiatives/comprehensive-primary-care-initiative/ (cited June 18, 2015).
228. Cahalin, L.P., et al. Current trends in reducing cardiovascular risk factors in the United States: focus on worksite health and wellness. *Prog Cardiovasc Dis*, 2014; 56(5): 476–83.
229. Goetzel, R.Z. Do prevention or treatment services save money? The wrong debate. *Health Aff* (Millwood), 2009; 28(1): 37–41.
230. James, J. Workplace wellness programs (updated). Health Affairs health policy briefs 2013. Available from http://www.healthaffairs.org/healthpolicybriefs/brief.php?brief_id=93 (cited November 17, 2014).

Index